Virtual Clinical Excursions—General Hospital

for

deWit:
Fundamental Concepts and Skills for Nursing,
3rd Edition

Virtual Clinical Excursions—General Hospital

for

deWit:
Fundamental Concepts and Skills for Nursing,
3rd Edition

prepared by

Kim Cooper, RN, MSN
Ivy Tech Community College
Terre Haute, Indiana

software developed by

Wolfsong Informatics, LLC
Tucson, Arizona

SAUNDERS
ELSEVIER

SAUNDERS
ELSEVIER

11830 Westline Industrial Dr.
St. Louis, Missouri 63146

VIRTUAL CLINICAL EXCURSIONS—GENERAL HOSPITAL FOR
DEWIT: FUNDAMENTAL CONCEPTS AND SKILLS FOR NURSING,
THIRD EDITION

ISBN: 978-1-4160-6224-0

Copyright © 2009, 2006 by Saunders, an imprint of Elsevier Inc.

ISBN: 978-1-4160-6224-0

Editor: *Jeff Downing*
Associate Developmental Editor: *Danny Witzofsky*
Project Manager: *Tracey Schriefer*
Book Production Manager: *Gayle May*

Printed in the United States of America

Last digit is the print number: 9 8 7 6 5 4 3

Working together to grow
libraries in developing countries

www.elsevier.com | www.bookaid.org | www.sabre.org

ELSEVIER   BOOK AID International   Sabre Foundation

*Workbook
prepared by*

Kim Cooper, RN, MSN
Ivy Tech Community College
Terre Haute, Indiana

Textbook

Susan C. deWit, MSN, RN, CNS, PHN
Formerly, Instructor of Nursing
El Centro College
Dallas, Texas

Contents

Table of Contents
deWit:
Fundamental Concepts and Skills for Nursing, 3rd Edition

Getting Started

GETTING SET UP

■ MINIMUM SYSTEM REQUIREMENTS

WINDOWS®

Windows Vista™, XP, 2000 (Recommend Windows XP/2000)
Pentium® III processor (or equivalent) @ 600 MHz (Recommend 800 MHz or better)
256 MB of RAM (Recommend 1 GB or more for Windows Vista)
800 x 600 screen size (Recommend 1024 x 768)
Thousands of colors
12x CD-ROM drive
Soundblaster 16 soundcard compatibility
Stereo speakers or headphones

Note: Windows Vista and XP require administrator privileges for installation.

MACINTOSH®

MAC OS X (10.2 or higher)
Apple Power PC G3 @ 500 MHz or better
128 MB of RAM (Recommend 256 MB or more)
800 x 600 screen size (Recommend 1024 x 768)
Thousands of colors
12x CD-ROM drive
Stereo speakers or headphones

1

■ INSTALLATION INSTRUCTIONS

WINDOWS

1. Insert the *Virtual Clinical Excursions—General Hospital* CD-ROM.
2. The setup screen should appear automatically if the current product is not already installed. Windows Vista users may be asked to authorize additional security prompts.
3. Follow the onscreen instructions during the setup process.

   If the setup screen does *not* appear automatically (and *Virtual Clinical Excursions—General Hospital* has not been installed already):
   a. Click the **My Computer** icon on your desktop or on your Start menu.
   b. Double-click on your CD-ROM drive.
   c. If installation does not start at this point:
      (1) Click the **Start** icon on the taskbar and select the **Run** option.
      (2) Type d:\setup.exe (where "d:\" is your CD-ROM drive) and press **OK**.
      (3) Follow the onscreen instructions for installation.

MACINTOSH

1. Insert the *Virtual Clinical Excursions—General Hospital* CD in the CD-ROM drive. The disk icon will appear on your desktop.

2. Double-click on the disk icon.

3. Double-click on the GENERAL-HOSPITAL_MAC run file.

Note: Virtual Clinical Excursions—General Hospital for Macintosh does not have an installation setup and can only be run directly from the CD.

■ HOW TO USE VIRTUAL CLINICAL EXCURSIONS—GENERAL HOSPITAL

WINDOWS

1. Double-click on the *Virtual Clinical Excursions—General Hospital* icon located on your desktop.
2. Or navigate to the program via the Windows Start menu.

Note: If your computer uses Windows Vista, right-click on the desktop shortcut and choose **Properties**. In the Compatability Mode, check the box for "Run as Administrator." Below is a screen capture to show what this looks like.

MACINTOSH

1. Insert the *Virtual Clinical Excursions—General Hospital* CD in the CD-ROM drive. The disk icon will appear on your desktop.

2. Double-click on the disk icon.

3. Double-click on the GENERAL-HOSPITAL_MAC run file.

■ SCREEN SETTINGS

For best results, your computer monitor resolution should be set at a minimum of 800 x 600. The number of colors displayed should be set to "thousands or higher" (High Color or 16 bit) or "millions of colors" (True Color or 24 bit).

Windows

1. From the **Start** menu, select **Control Panel** (on some systems, you will first go to **Settings**, then to **Control Panel**).
2. Double-click on the **Display** icon.
3. Click on the **Settings** tab.
4. Under **Screen resolution** use the slider bar to select **800 by 600 pixels**.
5. Access the **Colors** drop-down menu by clicking on the down arrow.
6. Select **High Color (16 bit)** or **True Color (24 bit)**.
7. Click on **OK**.
8. You may be asked to verify the setting changes. Click **Yes**.
9. You may be asked to restart your computer to accept the changes. Click **Yes**.

Macintosh

1. Select the **Monitors** control panel.
2. Select **800 x 600** (or similar) from the **Resolution** area.
3. Select **Thousands** or **Millions** from the **Color Depth** area.

■ WEB BROWSERS

Supported web browsers include Microsoft Internet Explorer (IE) version 6.0 or higher and Mozilla Firefox version 2.0 or higher. The supported browser for Macs running OS X is Mozilla Firefox.

If you use America Online® (AOL) for web access, you will need AOL version 4.0 or higher and one of the browsers listed above. Do not use earlier versions of AOL with earlier versions of IE, because you will have difficulty accessing many features.

For best results with AOL:
- Connect to the Internet using AOL version 4.0 or higher.
- Open a private chat within AOL (this allows the AOL client to remain open, without asking whether you wish to disconnect while minimized).
- Minimize AOL.
- Launch a recommended browser.

■ TECHNICAL SUPPORT

Technical support for this product is available between 7:30 a.m. and 7 p.m. (CST), Monday through Friday. Before calling, be sure that your computer meets the minimum system requirements to run this software. Inside the United States and Canada, call 1-800-692-9010. Outside North America, call 314-872-8370. You may also fax your questions to 314-523-4932 or contact Technical Support through e-mail: technical.support@elsevier.com.

Trademarks: Windows, Macintosh, Pentium, and America Online are registered trademarks.

Copyright © 2009 by Mosby, Inc., an affiliate of Elsevier Inc.

All rights reserved. No part of this product may be reproduced or transmitted in any form or by any means, electronic or mechanical, including input or storage in any information system, without written permission from the publisher.

ACCESSING *Virtual Clinical Excursions—General Hospital* FROM EVOLVE ————————————————————————

The product you have purchased is part of the Evolve family of online courses and learning resources. Please read the following information thoroughly to get started.

To access your instructor's course on Evolve:

Your instructor will provide you with the username and password needed to access this specific course on the Evolve Learning System. Once you have received this information, please follow these instructions:

1. Go to the Evolve student page (http://evolve.elsevier.com/student).

2. Enter your username and password in the **Login to My Evolve** area and click the **Login** button.

3. You will be taken to your personalized **My Evolve** page, where the course will be listed in the **My Courses** module.

TECHNICAL REQUIREMENTS

To use an Evolve course, you will need access to a computer that is connected to the Internet and equipped with web browser software that supports frames. For optimal performance, it is recommended that you have speakers and use a high-speed Internet connection. However, slower dial-up modems (56 K minimum) are acceptable.

Whichever browser you use, the browser preferences must be set to enable cookies and JavaScript and the cache must be set to reload every time.

Enable Cookies

Browser	Steps
Internet Explorer (IE) 6.0 or higher	1. Select **Tools → Internet Options**. 2. Select **Privacy** tab. 3. Use the slider (slide down) to **Accept All Cookies**. 4. Click **OK**. -OR- 3. Click the **Advanced** button. 4. Click the check box next to **Override Automatic Cookie Handling**. 5. Click the **Accept** radio buttons under **First-party Cookies** and **Third-party Cookies**. 6. Click **OK**.
Mozilla Firefox 2.0 or higher	1. Select **Tools → Options**. 2. Select the **Privacy** icon. 3. Click to expand Cookies. 4. Select **Allow sites to set cookies**. 5. Click **OK**.

Set Cache to Always Reload a Page

Browser	Steps
Internet Explorer (IE) 6.0 or higher	1. Select **Tools → Internet Options**. 2. Select **General** tab. 3. Go to the **Temporary Internet Files** and click the **Settings** button. 4. Select the radio button for **Every visit to the page** and click **OK** when complete.
Mozilla Firefox 2.0 or higher	1. Select **Tools → Options**. 2. Select the **Privacy** icon. 3. Click to expand Cache. 4. Set the value to "**0**" in the **Use up to: __ MB of disk space for the cache** field. 5. Click **OK**.

Plug-Ins

 Adobe Acrobat Reader—With the free Acrobat Reader software, you can view and print Adobe PDF files. Many Evolve products offer student and instructor manuals, checklists, and more in this format!

Download at: http://www.adobe.com

 Apple QuickTime—Install this to hear word pronunciations, heart and lung sounds, and many other helpful audio clips within Evolve Online Courses!

Download at: http://www.apple.com

 Adobe Flash Player—This player will enhance your viewing of many Evolve web pages, as well as educational short-form to long-form animation within the Evolve Learning System!

Download at: http://www.adobe.com

 Adobe Shockwave Player—Shockwave is best for viewing the many interactive learning activities within Evolve Online Courses!

Download at: http://www.adobe.com

 Microsoft Word Viewer—With this viewer, Microsoft Word users can share documents with those who don't have Word, and users without Word can open and view Word documents. Many Evolve products have testbank, student and instructor manuals, and other documents available for downloading and viewing on your own computer!

Download at: http://www.microsoft.com

 Microsoft PowerPoint Viewer—With this viewer, you can access PowerPoint 97, 2000, and 2002 presentations even if you don't have PowerPoint. Many Evolve products have slides available for downloading and viewing on your own computer!

Download at: http://www.microsoft.com

SUPPORT INFORMATION

Live phone support is available to customers in the United States and Canada at **800-401-9962** from 7:30 a.m. to 7 p.m. (CST), Monday through Friday. Support is also available through email at evolve-support@elsevier.com.

Online 24/7 support can be accessed on the Evolve website (http://evolve.elsevier.com). Resources include:

- Guided tours
- Tutorials
- Frequently asked questions (FAQs)
- Online copies of course user guides
- And much more!

A QUICK TOUR

Welcome to *Virtual Clinical Excursions—General Hospital*, a virtual hospital setting in which you can work with multiple complex patient simulations and also learn to access and evaluate the information resources that are essential for high-quality patient care. The virtual hospital, Pacific View Regional Hospital, has realistic architecture and access to patient rooms, a Nurses' Station, and a Medication Room.

■ BEFORE YOU START

Make sure you have your textbook nearby when you use the *Virtual Clinical Excursions— General Hospital* CD. You will want to consult topic areas in your textbook frequently while working with the CD and using this workbook.

■ HOW TO SIGN IN

- Enter your name on the Student Nurse identification badge.
- Next, specify the floor on which you will work by clicking the down arrow next to **Select Floor**. For this quick tour, choose **Medical-Surgical**.
- Now click the down arrow next to **Select Period of Care**. This drop-down menu gives you four periods of care from which to choose. In Periods of Care 1 through 3, you can actively engage in patient assessment, entry of data in the electronic patient record (EPR), and medication administration. Period of Care 4 presents the day in review. Highlight and click the appropriate period of care. (For this quick tour, choose **Period of Care 1: 0730-0815**.)
- Click **Go**. This takes you to the Patient List screen (see example on page 11). Note that the virtual time is provided in the box at the lower left corner of the screen (0730, since we chose Period of Care 1).

Note: If you choose to work during Period of Care 4: 1900-2000, the Patient List screen is skipped since you are not able to visit patients or administer medications during the shift. Instead, you are taken directly to the Nurses' Station, where the records of all the patients on the floor are available for your review.

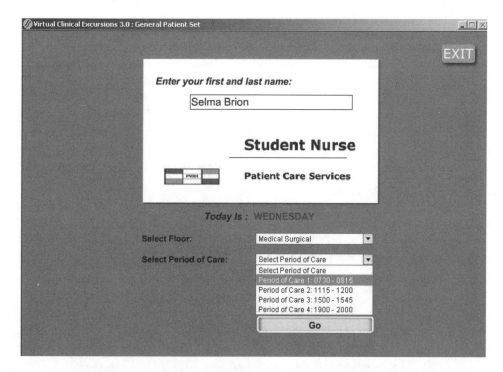

■ **PATIENT LIST**

MEDICAL-SURGICAL UNIT

Harry George (Room 401)
Osteomyelitis—A 54-year-old Caucasian male admitted from a homeless shelter with an infected leg. He has complications of type 2 diabetes mellitus, alcohol abuse, nicotine addiction, poor pain control, and complex psychosocial issues.

Jacquline Catanazaro (Room 402)
Asthma—A 45-year-old Caucasian female admitted with an acute asthma exacerbation and suspected pneumonia. She has complications of chronic schizophrenia, noncompliance with medication therapy, obesity, and herniated disc.

Piya Jordan (Room 403)
Bowel obstruction—A 68-year-old Asian female admitted with a colon mass and suspected adenocarcinoma. She undergoes a right hemicolectomy. This patient's complications include atrial fibrillation, hypokalemia, and symptoms of meperidine toxicity.

Clarence Hughes (Room 404)
Degenerative joint disease—A 73-year-old African-American male admitted for a left total knee replacement. His preparations for discharge are complicated by the development of a pulmonary embolus and the need for ongoing intravenous therapy.

Pablo Rodriguez (Room 405)
Metastatic lung carcinoma—A 71-year-old Hispanic male admitted with symptoms of dehydration and malnutrition. He has chronic pain secondary to multiple subcutaneous skin nodules and psychosocial concerns related to family issues with his approaching death.

Patricia Newman (Room 406)
Pneumonia—A 61-year-old Caucasian female admitted with worsening pulmonary function and an acute respiratory infection. Her chronic emphysema is complicated by heavy smoking, hypertension, and malnutrition. She needs access to community resources such as a smoking cessation program and meal assistance.

SKILLED NURSING UNIT

William Jefferson (Room 501)
Alzheimer's disease—A 75-year-old African-American male admitted for stabilization of type 2 diabetes and hypertension following a recent acute care admission for a urinary tract infection and sepsis. His complications include episodes of acute delirium and a history of osteoarthritis.

Kathryn Doyle (Room 503)
Rehabilitation post left hip replacement—A 79-year-old Caucasian female admitted following a complicated recovery from an ORIF. She is experiencing symptoms of malnutrition and depression due to unstable family dynamics, placing her at risk for elder abuse.

Goro Oishi (Room 505)
Hospice care—A 66-year-old Asian male admitted following an acute care admission for an intracerebral hemorrhage and resulting coma. Family-staff interactions provide opportunities to explore death and dying issues related to conflict about advanced life support and cultural and religious differences.

OBSTETRICS UNIT

Dorothy Grant (Room 201)
30-week intrauterine pregnancy—A 25-year-old multipara admitted with abdominal trauma following a domestic violence incident. Her complications include preterm labor and extensive social issues such as acquiring safe housing for her family upon discharge.

■ HOW TO SELECT A PATIENT

- You can choose one or more patients to work with from the Patient List by checking the box to the left of the patient name(s). For this quick tour, select Piya Jordan and Pablo Rodriguez. (In order to receive a scorecard for a patient, the patient must be selected before proceeding to the Nurses' Station.)
- Click on **Get Report** to the right of the medical records number (MRN) to view a summary of the patient's care during the 12-hour period before your arrival on the unit.
- After reviewing the report, click on **Go to Nurses' Station** in the right lower corner to begin your care. (*Note:* If you have been assigned to care for multiple patients, you can click on **Return to Patient List** to select and review the report for each additional patient before going to the Nurses' Station.)

Note: Even though the Patient List is initially skipped when you sign in to work for Period of Care 4, you can still access this screen if you wish to review the shift report for any of the patients. To do so, simply click on **Patient List** near the top left corner of the Nurses' Station (or click on the clipboard to the left of the Kardex). Then click on **Get Report** for the patient(s) whose care you are reviewing. This may be done during any period of care.

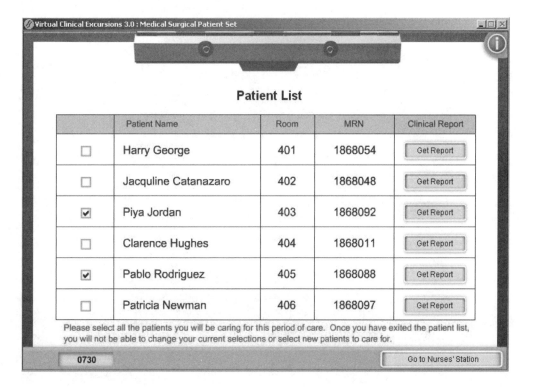

■ HOW TO FIND A PATIENT'S RECORDS

NURSES' STATION

Within the Nurses' Station, you will see:

1. A clipboard that contains the patient list for that floor.
2. A chart rack with patient charts labeled by room number, a notebook labeled Kardex, and a notebook labeled MAR (Medication Administration Record).
3. A desktop computer with access to the Electronic Patient Record (EPR).
4. A tool bar across the top of the screen that can also be used to access the Patient List, EPR, Chart, MAR, and Kardex. This tool bar is also accessible from each patient's room.
5. A Drug Guide containing information about the medications you are able to administer to your patients.
6. A tool bar across the bottom of the screen that can be used to access the Floor Map, patient rooms, Medication Room, and Drug Guide.

As you run your cursor over an item, it will be highlighted. To select, simply double-click on the item. As you use these resources, you will always be able to return to the Nurses' Station by clicking on the **Return to Nurses' Station** bar located in the right lower corner of your screen.

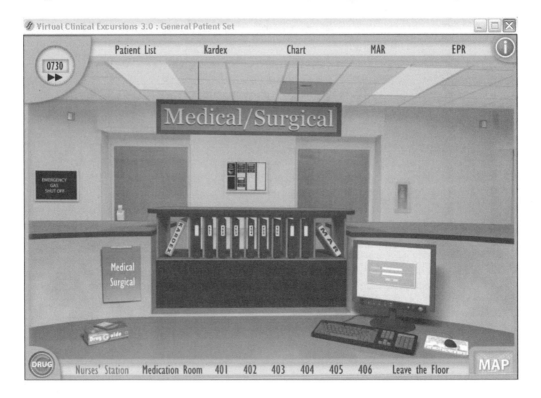

MEDICATION ADMINISTRATION RECORD (MAR)

The MAR icon located on the tool bar at the top of your screen accesses current 24-hour medications for each patient. Click on the icon and the MAR will open. (*Note:* You can also access the MAR by clicking on the MAR notebook on the far right side of the book rack in the center of the screen.) Within the MAR, tabs on the right side of the screen allow you to select patients by room number. Be careful to make sure you select the correct tab number for *your* patient rather than simply reading the first record that appears after the MAR opens. Each MAR sheet lists the following:

- Medications
- Route and dosage of each medication
- Times of administration of each medication

Note: The MAR changes each day. Expired MARs are stored in the patients' charts.

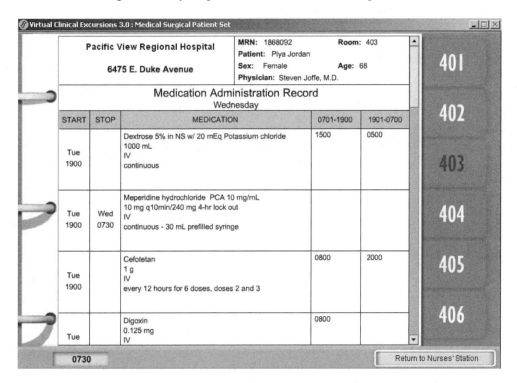

CHARTS

To access patient charts, either click on the **Chart** icon at the top of your screen or anywhere within the chart rack in the center of the Nurses' Station screen. When the close-up view appears, the individual charts are labeled by room number. To open a chart, click on the room number of the patient whose chart you wish to review. The patient's name and allergies will appear on the left side of the screen, along with a list of tabs on the right side of the screen, allowing you to view the following data:

- Allergies
- Physician's Orders
- Physician's Notes
- Nurse's Notes
- Laboratory Reports
- Diagnostic Reports
- Surgical Reports
- Consultations

- Patient Education
- History and Physical
- Nursing Admission
- Expired MARs
- Consents
- Mental Health
- Admissions
- Emergency Department

Information appears in real time. The entries are in reverse chronologic order, so use the down arrow at the right side of each chart page to scroll down to view previous entries. Flip from tab to tab to view multiple data fields or click on **Return to Nurses' Station** in the lower right corner of the screen to exit the chart.

Electronic Patient Record (EPR)

The EPR can be accessed from the computer in the Nurses' Station or from the EPR icon located in the tool bar at the top of your screen. To access a patient's EPR:
- Click on either the computer screen or the **EPR** icon.
- Your username and password are automatically filled in.
- Click on **Login** to enter the EPR.
- *Note:* Like the MAR, the EPR is arranged numerically. Thus when you enter, you are initially shown the records of the patient in the lowest room number on the floor. To view the correct data for *your* patient, remember to select the correct room number, using the drop-down menu for the Patient field at the top left corner of the screen.

The EPR used in Pacific View Regional Hospital represents a composite of commercial versions being used in hospitals. You can access the EPR:
- to review existing data for a patient (by room number).
- to enter data you collect while working with a patient.

The EPR is updated daily, so no matter what day or part of a shift you are working, there will be a current EPR with the patient's data from the past days of the current hospital stay. This type of simulated EPR allows you to examine how data for different attributes have changed over time, as well as to examine data for all of a patient's attributes at a particular time. The EPR is fully functional (as it is in a real-life hospital). You can enter such data as blood pressure, breath sounds, and certain treatments. The EPR will not, however, allow you to enter data for a previous time period. Use the arrows at the bottom of the screen to move forward and backward in time.

Patient: 403	Category: Vital Signs			0732

Name: Piya Jordan	Wed 0630	Wed 0700	Wed 0715	Code Meanings	
PAIN: LOCATION		OS		A	Abdomen
PAIN: RATING		5		Ar	Arm
PAIN: CHARACTERISTICS		C		B	Back
PAIN: VOCAL CUES		VC3		C	Chest
PAIN: FACIAL CUES		FC1		Ft	Foot
PAIN: BODILY CUES				H	Head
PAIN: SYSTEM CUES				Hd	Hand
PAIN: FUNCTIONAL EFFECTS				L	Left
PAIN: PREDISPOSING FACTORS				Lg	Leg
PAIN: RELIEVING FACTORS				Lw	Lower
PCA		P		N	Neck
TEMPERATURE (F)		99.6		NN	See Nurses notes
TEMPERATURE (C)				OS	Operative site
MODE OF MEASUREMENT		Ty		Or	See Physicians orders
SYSTOLIC PRESSURE		110		PN	See Progress notes
DIASTOLIC PRESSURE		70		R	Right
BP MODE OF MEASUREMENT		NIBP		Up	Upper
HEART RATE		104			
RESPIRATORY RATE		18			
SpO2 (%)		95			
BLOOD GLUCOSE					
WEIGHT					
HEIGHT					

At the top of the EPR screen, you can choose patients by their room numbers. In addition, you have access to 17 different categories of patient data. To change patients or data categories, click the down arrow to the right of the room number or category.

The categories of patient data in the EPR as as follows:

- Vital Signs
- Respiratory
- Cardiovascular
- Neurologic
- Gastrointestinal
- Excretory
- Musculoskeletal
- Integumentary
- Reproductive
- Psychosocial
- Wounds and Drains
- Activity
- Hygiene and Comfort
- Safety
- Nutrition
- IV
- Intake and Output

Remember, each hospital selects its own codes. The codes used in the EPR at Pacific View Regional Hospital may be different from ones you have seen in your clinical rotations. Take some time to acquaint yourself with the codes. Within the Vital Signs category, click on any item in the left column (e.g., Pain: Characteristics). In the far-right column, you will see a list of code meanings for the possible findings and/or descriptors for that assessment area.

You will use the codes to record the data you collect as you work with patients. Click on the box in the last time column to the right of any item and wait for the code meanings applicable to that entry to appear. Select the appropriate code to describe your assessment findings and type it in the box. (*Note:* If no cursor appears within the box, click on the box again until the blue shading disappears and the blinking cursor appears.) Once the data are typed in this box, they are entered into the patient's record for this period of care only.

To leave the EPR, click on **Exit EPR** in the bottom right corner of the screen.

■ VISITING A PATIENT

From the Nurses' Station, click on the room number of the patient you wish to visit (in the tool bar at the bottom of your screen). Once you are inside the room, you will see a still photo of your patient in the top left corner. To verify that this is the correct patient, click on the **Check Armband** icon to the right of the photo. The patient's identification data will appear. If you click on **Check Allergies** (the next icon to the right), a list of the patient's allergies (if any) will replace the photo.

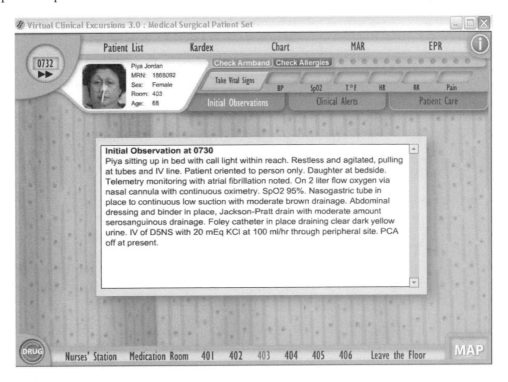

Also located in the patient's room are multiple icons you can use to assess the patient or the patient's medications. A virtual clock is provided in the upper left corner of the room to monitor your progress in real time. (*Note:* The fast-forward icon within the virtual clock will advance the time by 2-minute intervals when clicked.)

- The tool bar across the top of the screen allows you to check the **Patient List**, access the **EPR** to check or enter data, and view the patient's **Chart**, **MAR**, or **Kardex**.

- The **Take Vital Signs** icon allows you to measure the patient's up-to-the-minute blood pressure, oxygen saturation, temperature, heart rate, respiratory rate, and pain level.

- Each time you enter a patient's room, you are given an Initial Observation report to review (in the text box under the patient's photo). These notes are provided to give you a "look" at the patient as if you had just stepped into the room. You can also click on the **Initial Observations** icon to return to this box from other views within the patient's room. To the right of this icon is **Clinical Alerts**, a resource that allows you to make decisions about priority medication interventions based on emerging data collected in real time. Check this screen throughout your period of care to avoid missing critical information related to recently ordered or STAT medications.

- Clicking on **Patient Care** opens up three specific learning environments within the patient room: **Physical Assessment**, **Nurse-Client Interactions**, and **Medication Administration**.

- To perform a **Physical Assessment**, choose a body area (such as **Head & Neck**) from the column of yellow buttons. This activates a list of system subcategories for that body area (e.g., see **Sensory**, **Neurologic**, etc. in the green boxes). After you select the system you wish to evaluate, a brief description of the assessment findings will appear in a box to the right. A still photo provides a "snapshot" of how an assessment of this area might be done or what the finding might look like. For every body area, you can also click on **Equipment** on the right side of the screen.

- To the right of the Physical Assessment icon is **Nurse-Client Interactions**. Clicking on this icon will reveal the times and titles of any videos available for viewing. (*Note:* If the video you wish to see is not listed, this means you have not yet reached the correct virtual time to view that video. Check the virtual clock; you may return to access the video once its designated time has occurred—as long as you do so within the same period of care. Or you can click on the fast-forward icon within the virtual clock to advance the time by 2-minute intervals. You will then need to click again on **Patient Care** and **Nurse-Client Interactions** to refresh the screen.) To view a listed video, click on the white arrow to the right of the video title. Use the control buttons below the video to start, stop, pause, rewind, or fast-forward the action or to mute the sound.

- **Medication Administration** is the pathway that allows you to review and administer medications to a patient after you have prepared them in the Medication Room. This process is addressed further in the *How to Prepare Medications* section (pages 19-20) and in *Medications* (pages 26-30). For additional hands-on practice, see *Reducing Medication Errors* (pages 37-41).

■ HOW TO QUIT, CHANGE PATIENTS, CHANGE FLOORS, OR CHANGE PERIODS OF CARE

How to Quit: From most screens, you may click the **Leave the Floor** icon on the bottom tool bar to the right of the patient room numbers. (*Note:* From some screens, you will first need to click an **Exit** button or **Return to Nurses' Station** before clicking **Leave the Floor**.) When the Floor Menu appears, click **Exit** to leave the program.

How to Change Patients, Floors, or Periods of Care: To change patients, simply click on the new patient's room number. (You cannot receive a scorecard for a new patient, however, unless you have already selected that patient on the Patient List screen.) To change to a new period of care, to change floors, or to restart the virtual clock, click on **Leave the Floor** and then on **Restart the Program**.

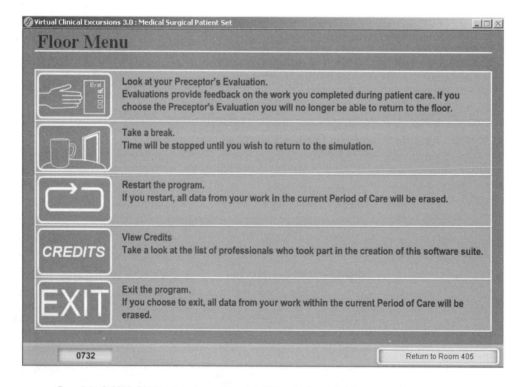

■ HOW TO PREPARE MEDICATIONS

From the Nurses' Station or the patient's room, you can access the Medication Room by clicking on the icon in the tool bar at the bottom of your screen to the left of the patient room numbers.

In the Medication Room you have access to the following (from left to right):

- A preparation area is located on the counter under the cabinets. To begin the medication preparation process, click on the tray on the counter or click on the **Preparation** icon at the top of the screen. The next screen leads you through a specific sequence (called the Preparation Wizard) to prepare medications one at a time for administration to a patient. However, no medication has been selected at this time. We will do this while working with a patient in *A Detailed Tour*. To exit this screen, click on **View Medication Room**.

- To the right of the cabinets (and above the refrigerator), IV storage bins are provided. Click on the bins themselves or on the **IV Storage** icon at the top of the screen. The bins are labeled **Microinfusion**, **Small Volume**, and **Large Volume**. Click on an individual bin to see a list of its contents. If you needed to prepare an IV medication at this time, you could click on the medication and its label would appear to the right under the patient's name. (*Note:* You can **Open** and **Close** any medication label by clicking the appropriate icon.) Next, you would click **Put Medication on Tray**. If you ever change your mind or decide that you have put the incorrect medication on the tray, you can reverse your actions by highlighting the medication on the tray and then clicking **Put Medication in Bin**. Click **Close Bin** in the right bottom corner to exit. **View Medication Room** brings you back to a full view of the entire room.

- A refrigerator is located under the IV storage bins to hold any medications that must be stored below room temperature. Click on the refrigerator door or on the **Refrigerator** icon at the top of the screen. Then click on the close-up view of the door to access the medications. When you are finished, click **Close Door** and then **View Medication Room**.

- To prepare controlled substances, click the **Automated System** icon at the top of the screen or click the computer monitor located to the right of the IV storage bins. A login screen will appear; your name and password are automatically filled in. Click **Login**. Select the patient for whom you wish to access medications; then select the correct medication drawer to open (they are stored alphabetically). Click **Open Drawer**, highlight the proper medication, and choose **Put Medication on Tray**. When you are finished, click **Close Drawer** and then **View Medication Room**.

- Next to the Automated System is a set of drawers identified by patient room number. To access these, click on the drawers or on the **Unit Dosage** icon at the top of the screen. This provides a close-up view of the drawers. To open a drawer, click on the room number of the patient you are working with. Next, click on the medication you would like to prepare for the patient, and a label will appear, listing the medication strength, units, and dosage per unit. To exit, click **Close Drawer**; then click **View Medication Room**.

At any time, you can learn about a medication you wish to prepare for a patient by clicking on the **Drug** icon in the bottom left corner of the medication room screen or by clicking the **Drug Guide** book on the counter to the right of the unit dosage drawers. The **Drug Guide** provides information about the medications commonly included in nursing drug handbooks. Nutritional supplements and maintenance intravenous fluid preparations are not included. Highlight a medication in the alphabetical list; relevant information about the drug will appear in the screen below. To exit, click **Return to Medication Room**.

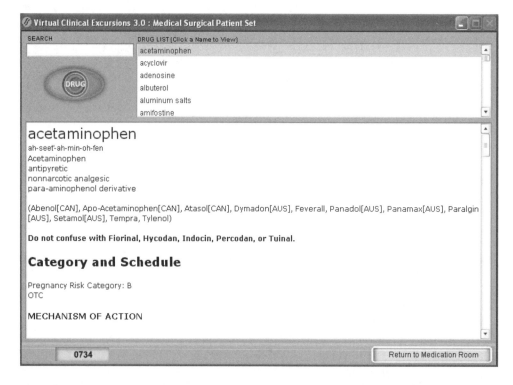

To access the MAR to review the medications ordered for a patient, click on the **MAR** icon located in the tool bar at the top of your screen and then click on the correct tab for your patient's room number. You may also click the **Review MAR** icon in the tool bar at the bottom of your screen from inside each medication storage area.

After you have chosen and prepared medications, go to the patient's room to administer them by clicking on the room number in the bottom tool bar. Inside the patient's room, click **Patient Care** and then **Medication Administration** and follow the proper administration sequence.

■ PRECEPTOR'S EVALUATIONS

When you have finished a session, click on **Leave the Floor** to go to the Floor Menu. At this point, you can click on the top icon (**Look at Your Preceptor's Evaluation**) to receive a score-card that provides feedback on the work you completed during patient care.

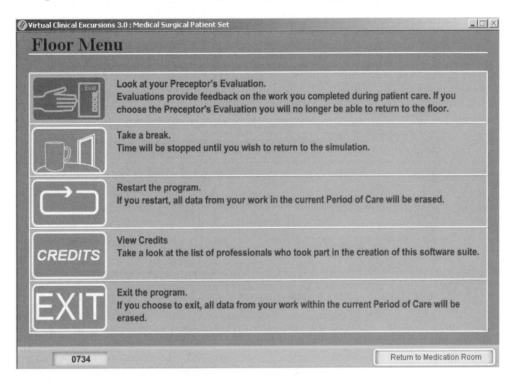

Evaluations are available for each patient you selected when you signed in for the current period of care. Click on the **Medication Scorecard** icon to see an example.

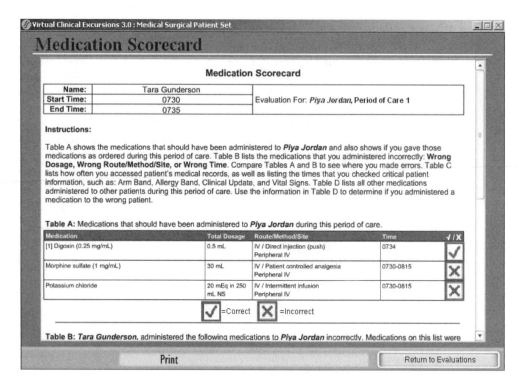

The scorecard compares the medications you administered to a patient during a period of care with what should have been administered. Table A lists the correct medications. Table B lists any medications that were administered incorrectly.

Remember, not every medication listed on the MAR should necessarily be given. For example, a patient might have an allergy to a drug that was ordered, or a medication might have been improperly transcribed to the MAR. Predetermined medication "errors" embedded within the program challenge you to exercise critical thinking skills and professional judgment when deciding to administer a medication, just as you would in a real hospital. Use all your available resources, such as the patient's chart and the MAR, to make your decision.

Table C lists the resources that were available to assist you in medication administration. It also documents whether and when you accessed these resources. For example, did you check the patient armband or perform a check of vital signs? If so, when?

You can click **Print** to get a copy of this report if needed. When you have finished reviewing the scorecard, click **Return to Evaluations** and then **Return to Menu**.

■ FLOOR MAP

To get a general sense of your location within the hospital, you can click on the **Map** icon found in the lower right corner of most of the screens in the *Virtual Clinical Excursions—General Hospital* program. (*Note:* If you are following this quick tour step by step, you will need to **Restart the Program** from the Floor Menu, sign in again, and go to the Nurses' Station to access the map.) When you click the **Map** icon, a floor map appears, showing the layout of the floor you are currently on, as well as a directory of the patients and services on that floor. As you move your cursor over the directory list, the location of each room is highlighted on the map (and vice versa). The floor map can be accessed from the Nurses' Station, Medication Room, and each patient's room.

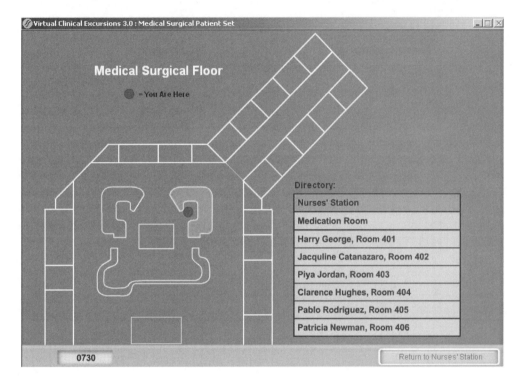

A DETAILED TOUR

If you wish to more thoroughly understand the capabilities of *Virtual Clinical Excursions—General Hospital*, take a detailed tour by completing the following section. During this tour, we will work with a specific patient to introduce you to all the different components and learning opportunities available within the software.

■ WORKING WITH A PATIENT

Sign in and select the Medical-Surgical Floor for Period of Care 1 (0730-0815). From the Patient List, select Piya Jordan and Pablo Rodriguez; however, do not go to the Nurses' Station yet.

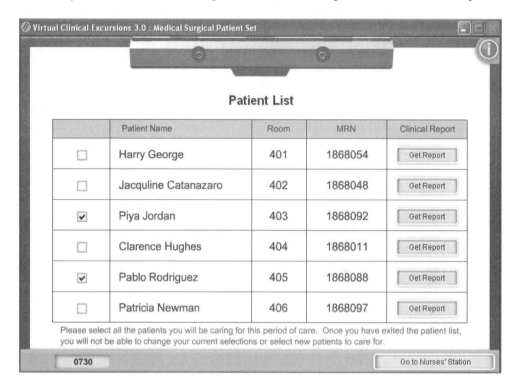

■ REPORT

In hospitals, when one shift ends and another begins, the outgoing nurse who attended a patient will give a verbal and sometimes a written summary of that patient's condition to the incoming nurse who will assume care for the patient. This summary is called a report and is an important source of data to provide an overview of a patient. Your first task is to get the clinical report on Piya Jordan. To do this, click **Get Report** in the far right column in this patient's row. From a brief review of this summary, identify the problems and areas of concern that you will need to address for this patient.

When you have finished noting any areas of concern, click on **Go to Nurses' Station**.

■ CHARTS

You can access Piya Jordan's chart from the Nurses' Station or from the patient's room (403). From the Nurses' Station, click on the chart rack or on the **Chart** icon in the tool bar at the top of your screen. Next, click on the chart labeled **403** to open the medical record for Piya Jordan. Click on the **Emergency Department** tab to view a record of why this patient was admitted.

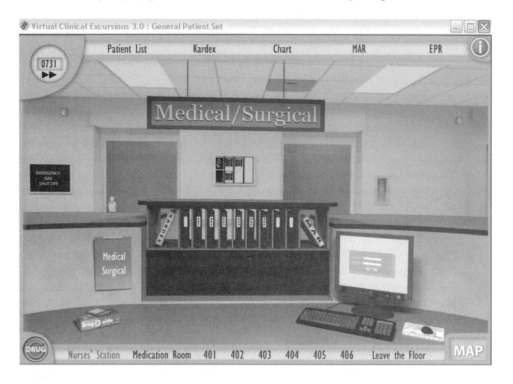

How many days has Piya Jordan been in the hospital?

What tests were done upon her arrival in the Emergency Department and why?

What was her reason for admission?

You should also click on **Surgical Reports** to learn what procedures were performed and when. Finally, review the **Nursing Admission** and **History and Physical** to learn about the health history of this patient. When you are done reviewing the chart, click **Return to Nurses' Station**.

■ **MEDICATIONS**

Open the Medication Administration Record (MAR) by clicking on the **MAR** icon in the tool bar at the top of your screen. *Remember:* The MAR automatically opens to the first occupied room number on the floor—which is not necessarily your patient's room number! Since you need to access Piya Jordan's MAR, click on tab **403** (her room number). Always make sure you are giving the *Right Drug to the Right Patient!*

Examine the list of medications ordered for Piya Jordan. In the table below, list the medications that need to be given during this period of care (0730-0815). For each medication, note the dosage, route, and time to be given.

Time	Medication	Dosage	Route

Click on **Return to Nurses' Station**. Next, click on **403** on the bottom tool bar and then verify that you are indeed in Piya Jordan's room. Select **Clinical Alerts** (the icon to the right of Initial Observations) to check for any emerging data that might affect your medication administration priorities. Next, go to the patient's chart (click on the **Chart** icon; then click on **403**). When the chart opens, select the **Physician's Orders** tab.

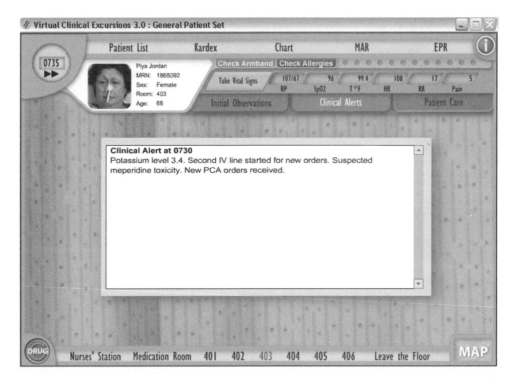

Review the orders. Have any new medications been ordered? Return to the MAR (click **Return to Room 403**; then click **MAR**). Verify that the new medications have been correctly transcribed to the MAR. Mistakes are sometimes made in the transcription process in the hospital setting, and it is sound practice to double-check any new order.

Are there any patient assessments you will need to perform before administering these medications? If so, return to Room 403 and click on **Patient Care** and then **Physical Assessment** to complete those assessments before proceeding.

Now click on the **Medication Room** icon in the tool bar at the bottom of your screen to locate and prepare the medications for Piya Jordan.

In the Medication Room, you must access the medications for Piya Jordan from the specific dispensing system in which each medication is stored. Locate each medication that needs to be given in this time period and click on **Put Medication on Tray** as appropriate. (*Hint:* Look in **Unit Dosage** drawer first.) When you are finished, click on **Close Drawer** and then on **View Medication Room**. Now click on the medication tray on the counter on the left side of the medication room screen to begin preparing the medications you have selected. (*Remember:* You can also click **Preparation** in the tool bar at the top of the screen.)

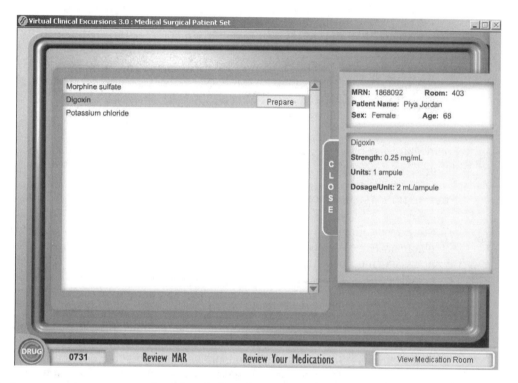

In the preparation area, you should see a list of the medications you put on the tray in the previous steps. Click on the first medication and then click **Prepare**. Follow the onscreen instructions of the Preparation Wizard, providing any data requested. As an example, let's follow the preparation process for digoxin, one of the medications due to be administered to Piya Jordan during this period of care. To begin, click to select **Digoxin**; then click **Prepare**. Now work through the Preparation Wizard sequence as detailed below:

Amount of medication in the ampule: 2 mL.
Enter the amount of medication you will draw up into a syringe: <u>**0.5**</u> mL.
Click **Next**.
Select the patient you wish to set aside the medication for: **Room 403, Piya Jordan**.
Click **Finish**.
Click **Return to Medication Room**.

Follow this same basic process for the other medications due to be administered to Piya Jordan during this period of care. (*Hint:* Look in **IV Storage** and **Automated System**.)

PREPARATION WIZARD EXCEPTIONS

- Some medications in *Virtual Clinical Excursions—General Hospital* are prepared by the pharmacy (e.g., IV antibiotics) and taken to the patient room as a whole. This is common practice in most hospitals.
- Blood products are not administered by students through the *Virtual Clinical Excursions—General Hospital* simulations since blood administration follows specific protocols not covered in this program.
- The *Virtual Clinical Excursions—General Hospital* simulations do not allow for mixing more than one type of medication, such as regular and Lente insulins, in the same syringe. In the clinical setting, when multiple types of insulin are ordered for a patient, the regular insulin is drawn up first, followed by the longer-acting insulin. Insulin is always administered in a special unit-marked syringe.

Now return to Room 403 (click on **403** on the bottom tool bar) to administer Piya Jordan's medications.

At any time during the medication administration process, you can perform a further review of systems, take vital signs, check information contained within the chart, or verify patient identity and allergies. Inside Piya Jordan's room, click **Take Vital Signs**. (*Note:* These findings change over time to reflect the temporal changes you would find in a patient similar to Piya Jordan.)

When you have gathered all the data you need, click on **Patient Care** and then select **Medication Administration**. Any medications you prepared in the previous steps should be listed on the left side of your screen. Let's continue the administration process with the digoxin ordered for Piya Jordan. Click to highlight **Digoxin** in the list of medications. Next, click on the down arrow to the right of **Select** and choose **Administer** from the drop-down menu. This will activate the Administration Wizard. Complete the Wizard sequence as follows:

- Route: **IV**
- Method: **Direct Injection**
- Site: **Peripheral IV**
- Click **Administer to Patient** arrow.
- Would you like to document this administration in the MAR? **Yes**
- Click **Finish** arrow.

Your selections are recorded by a tracking system and evaluated on a Medication Scorecard stored under Preceptor's Evaluations. This scorecard can be viewed, printed, and given to your instructor. To access the Preceptor's Evaluations, click on **Leave the Floor**. When the Floor Menu appears, select **Look at Your Preceptor's Evaluation**. Then click on **Medication Scorecard** inside the box with Piya Jordan's name (see example on the following page).

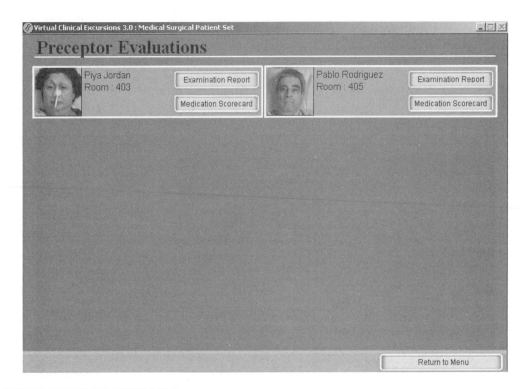

■ MEDICATION SCORECARD

- First, review Table A. Was digoxin given correctly? Did you give the other medications as ordered?
- Table B shows you which (if any) medications you gave incorrectly.
- Table C addresses the resources used for Piya Jordan. Did you access the patient's chart, MAR, EPR, or Kardex as needed to make safe medication administration decisions?
- Did you check the patient's armband to verify her identity? Did you check whether your patient had any known allergies to medications? Were vital signs taken?

When you have finished reviewing the scorecard, click **Return to Evaluations** and then **Return to Menu**.

■ VITAL SIGNS

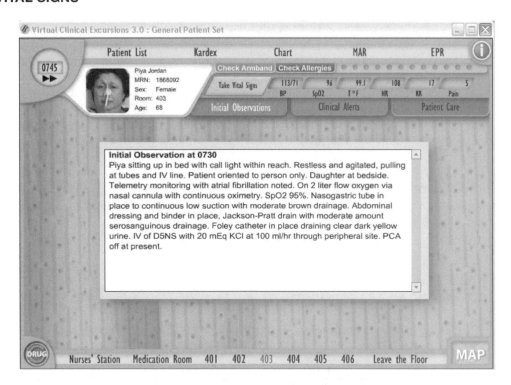

Vital signs, often considered the traditional "signs of life," include body temperature, heart rate, respiratory rate, blood pressure, oxygen saturation of the blood, and pain level.

Inside Piya Jordan's room, click **Take Vital Signs**. (*Note:* If you are following this detailed tour step by step, you will need to **Restart the Program** from the Floor Menu, sign in again, and navigate to Room 403.) Collect vital signs for this patient and record them below. Note the time at which you collected each of these data. (*Remember:* You can take vital signs at any time. The data change over time to reflect the temporal changes you would find in a patient similar to Piya Jordan.)

Vital Signs	Findings/Time
Blood pressure	
O$_2$ saturation	
Heart rate	
Respiratory rate	
Temperature	
Pain rating	

After you are done, click on the **EPR** icon located in the tool bar at the top of the screen. Your username and password are automatically provided. Click on **Login** to enter the EPR. To access Piya Jordan's records, click on the down arrow next to Patient and choose her room number, **403**. Select **Vital Signs** as the category. Next, in the empty time column on the far right, record the vital signs data you just collected in Piya Jordan's room. (*Note:* If you need help with this process, see page 16.) Now compare these findings with the data you collected earlier for this patient's vital signs. Use these earlier findings to establish a baseline for each of the vital signs.

  a. Are any of the data you collected significantly different from the baseline for a particular vital sign?

    Circle One: Yes   No

  b. If "Yes," which data are different?

■ PHYSICAL ASSESSMENT

After you have finished examining the EPR for vital signs, click **Exit EPR** to return to Room 403. Click **Patient Care** and then **Physical Assessment**. Think about the information you received in the report at the beginning of this shift, as well as what you may have learned about this patient from the chart. Based on this, what area(s) of examination should you pay most attention to at this time? Is there any equipment you should be monitoring? Conduct a physical assessment of the body areas and systems that you consider priorities for Piya Jordan. For example, select **Head & Neck**; then click on and assess **Sensory** and **Lymphatic**. Complete any other assessment(s) you think are necessary at this time. In the following table, record the data you collected during this examination.

Area of Examination	Findings
Head & Neck Sensory	
Head & Neck Lymphatic	

After you have finished collecting these data, return to the EPR. Compare the data that were already in the record with those you just collected.

    a.   Are any of the data you collected significantly different from the baselines for this patient?

       Circle One: Yes   No

    b.   If "Yes," which data are different?

■ **NURSE-CLIENT INTERACTIONS**

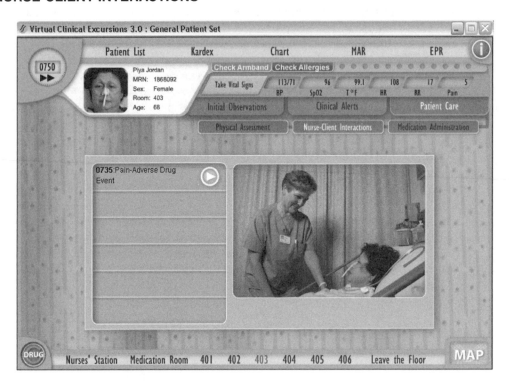

Click on **Patient Care** from inside Piya Jordan's room (403). Now click on **Nurse-Client Interactions** to access a short video titled **Pain—Adverse Drug Event**, which is available for viewing at or after 0735 (based on the virtual clock in the upper left corner of your screen; see *Note* below.). To begin the video, click on the white arrow next to its title. You will observe a nurse communicating with Piya Jordan and her daughter. There are many variations of nursing practice, some exemplifying "best" practice and some not. Note whether the nurse in this interaction displays professional behavior and compassionate care. Are her words congruent with what is going on with the patient? Does this interaction "feel right" to you? If not, how would you handle this situation differently? Explain.

Note: If the video you wish to view is not listed, this means you have not yet reached the correct virtual time to view that video. Check the virtual clock; you may return to access the video once its designated time has occurred—as long as you do so within the same period of care. Or you can click on the fast-forward icon within the virtual clock to advance the time by 2-minute intervals. You will then need to click again on **Patient Care** and **Nurse-Client Interactions** to refresh the screen.

At least one Nurse-Client Interactions video is available during each period of care. Viewing these videos can help you learn more about what is occurring with a patient at a certain time and also prompt you to discern between nurse communications that are ideal and those that need improvement. Compassionate care and the ability to communicate clearly are essential components of delivering quality nursing care, and it is during your clinical time that you will begin to refine these skills.

■ COLLECTING AND EVALUATING DATA

Each of the activities you perform in the Patient Care environment generates a significant amount of assessment data. Remember that after you collect data, you can record your findings in the EPR. You can also review the EPR, patient's chart, videos, and MAR at any time. You will get plenty of practice collecting and then evaluating data in context of the patient's course.

Now, here's an important question for you:

> Did the previous sequence of exercises provide the most efficient way to assess Piya Jordan?

For example, you went to the patient's room to get vital signs, then back to the EPR to enter data and compare your findings with extant data. Next, you went back to the patient's room to do a physical examination, then again back to the EPR to enter and review data. If this back-and-forth process of data collection and recording seemed inefficient, remember the following:

- Plan all of your nursing activities to maximize efficiency, while at the same time optimizing the quality of patient care. (Think about what data you might need before performing certain tasks. For example, do you need to check a heart rate before administering a cardiac medication or check an IV site before starting an infusion?)

- You collect a tremendous amount of data when you work with a patient. Very few people can accurately remember all these data for more than a few minutes. Develop efficient assessment skills, and record data as soon as possible after collecting them.

- Assessment data are only the starting point for the nursing process.

Make a clear distinction between these first exercises and how you actually provide nursing care. These initial exercises were designed to involve you actively in the use of different software components. This workbook focuses on sensible practices for implementing the nursing process in ways that ensure the highest-quality care of patients.

Most important, remember that a human being changes through time, and that these changes include both the physical and psychosocial facets of a person as a living organism. Think about this for a moment. Some patients may change physically in a very short time (a patient with emerging myocardial infarction) or more slowly (a patient with a chronic illness). Patients' overall physical and psychosocial conditions may improve or deteriorate. They may have effective coping skills and familial support, or they may feel alone and full of despair. In fact, each individual is a complex mix of physical and psychosocial elements, and at least some of these elements usually change through time.

Thus it is crucial that you *DO NOT* think of the nursing process as a simple one-time, five-step procedure consisting of assessment, nursing diagnosis, planning, implementation, and evaluation. Rather, the nursing process should be utilized as a creative and systematic approach to delivering nursing care. Furthermore, because all living organisms are constantly changing, we must apply the nursing process over and over. Each time we follow the nursing process for an individual patient, we refine our understanding of that patient's physical and psychosocial conditions based on collection and analysis of many different types of data. *Virtual Clinical Excursions—General Hospital* will help you develop both the creativity and the systematic approach needed to become a nurse who is equipped to deliver the highest-quality care to all patients.

REDUCING MEDICATION ERRORS

Earlier in this detailed tour, you learned the basic steps of medication preparation and administration. The following simulations will allow you to practice those skills further—with an increased emphasis on reducing medication errors by using the Medication Scorecard to evaluate your work.

Sign in to work on the Medical-Surgical Floor at Pacific View Regional Hospital for Period of Care 1. (*Note:* If you are already working with another patient or during another period of care, click on **Leave the Floor** and then **Restart the Program**; then sign in.)

From the Patient List, select Clarence Hughes. Then click on **Go to Nurses' Station**. Complete the following steps to prepare and administer medications to Clarence Hughes.

- Click on **Medication Room**.
- Click on **MAR** and then on tab **404** to determine prn medications that have been ordered for Clarence Hughes. (*Note:* You may click on **Review MAR** at any time to verify the correct medication order. Always remember to check the patient name on the MAR to make sure you have the correct patient's record—you must click on the correct room number tab within the MAR.) Click on **Return to Medication Room** after reviewing the correct MAR.
- Click on **Unit Dosage** (or on the Unit Dosage cabinet); from the close-up view, click on drawer **404**.
- Select the medications you would like to administer. After each selection, click **Put Medication on Tray**. When you are finished selecting medications, click **Close Drawer** and then **View Medication Room**.
- Click **Automated System** (or on the Automated System unit itself). Click **Login**.
- On the next screen, specify the correct patient and drawer location.
- Select the medication you would like to administer and click **Put Medication on Tray**. Repeat this process if you wish to administer other medications from the Automated System.
- When you are finished, click **Close Drawer** and **View Medication Room**.
- From the Medication Room, click **Preparation** (or on the preparation tray).
- From the list of medications on your tray, highlight the correct medication to administer and click **Prepare**.
- This activates the Preparation Wizard. Supply any requested information; then click **Next**.
- Now select the correct patient to receive this medication and click **Finish**.
- Repeat the previous three steps until all medications that you want to administer are prepared.
- You can click on **Review Your Medications** and then on **Return to Medication Room** when ready. Once you are back in the Medication Room, go directly to Clarence Hughes' room by clicking on **404** at the bottom of the screen.
- Inside the patient's room, administer the medication, utilizing the five rights of medication administration. After you have collected the appropriate assessment data and are ready for administration, click **Patient Care** and then **Medication Administration**. Verify that the correct patient and medication(s) appear in the left-hand window. Highlight the first medication you wish to administer; then click the down arrow next to Select. From the drop-down menu, select **Administer** and complete the Administration Wizard by providing any information requested. When the Wizard stops asking for information, click **Administer to Patient**. Specify **Yes** when asked whether this administration should be recorded in the MAR. Finally, click **Finish**.

■ **SELF-EVALUATION**

Now let's see how you did during your medication administration!

• Click on **Leave the Floor** at the bottom of your screen. From the Floor Menu, select **Look at Your Preceptor's Evaluation**. Then click **Medication Scorecard**.

The following exercises will help you identify medication errors, investigate possible reasons for these errors, and reduce or prevent medication errors in the future.

1. Start by examining Table A. These are the medications you should have given to Clarence Hughes during this period of care. If each of the medications in Table A has a ✓ by it, then you made no errors. Congratulations!

If any medication has an X by it, then you made one or more medication errors.

Compare Tables A and B to determine which of the following types of errors you made: Wrong Dose, Wrong Route/Method/Site, or Wrong Time. Follow these steps:
   a. Find medications in Table A that were given incorrectly.
   b. Now see if those same medications are in Table B, which shows what you actually administered to Clarence Hughes.
   c. Comparing Tables A and B, match the Strength, Dose, Route/Method/Site, and Time for each medication you administered incorrectly.
   d. Then, using the form below, list the medications given incorrectly and mark the errors you made for each medication.

Medication	Strength	Dosage	Route	Method	Site	Time
	❑	❑	❑	❑	❑	❑
	❑	❑	❑	❑	❑	❑
	❑	❑	❑	❑	❑	❑
	❑	❑	❑	❑	❑	❑

2. To help you reduce future medication errors, consider the following list of possible reasons for errors.

• Did not check drug against MAR for correct patient, correct date, correct time, correct drug, and correct dose.
• Did not check drug dose against MAR three times.
• Did not open the unit dose package in the patient's room.
• Did not correctly identify the patient using two identifiers.
• Did not administer the drug on time.
• Did not verify patient allergies.
• Did not check the patient's current condition or vital sign parameters.
• Did not consider why the patient would be receiving this drug.
• Did not question why the drug was in the patient's drawer.
• Did not check the physician's order and/or check with the pharmacist when there was a question about the drug or dose.
• Did not verify that no adverse effects had occurred from a previous dose.

Based on the list of possibilities you just reviewed, determine how you made each error and record the reason in the form below:

Medication	Reason for Error

3. Look again at Table B. Are there medications listed that are not in Table A? If so, you gave a medication to Clarence Hughes that he should not have received. Complete the following exercises to help you understand how such an error might have been made.

   a. Perhaps you gave a medication that was on Clarence Hughes' MAR for this period of care, without recognizing that a change had occurred in the patient's condition, which should have caused you to reconsider. Review patient records as necessary and complete the following form:

Medication	Possible Reasons Not to Give This Medication

   b. Another possibility is that you gave Clarence Hughes a medication that should have been given at a different time. Check his MAR and complete the form below to determine whether you made a Wrong Time error:

Medication	Given to Clarence Hughes at What Time	Should Have Been Given at What Time

c. Maybe you gave another patient's medication to Clarence Hughes. In this case, you made a Wrong Patient error. Check the MARs of other patients and use the form below to determine whether you made this type of error:

Medication	Given to Clarence Hughes	Should Have Been Given to

4. The Medication Scorecard provides some other interesting sources of information. For example, if there is a medication selected for Clarence Hughes but it was not given to him, there will be an X by that medication in Table A, but it will not appear in Table B. In that case, you might have given this medication to some other patient, which is another type of Wrong Patient error. To investigate further, look at Table D, which lists the medications you gave to other patients. See whether you can find any medications ordered for Clarence Hughes that were given to another patient by mistake. However, before you make any decisions, be sure to cross-check the MAR for other patients because the same medication may have been ordered for multiple patients. Use the following form to record your findings:

Medication	Should Have Been Given to Clarence Hughes	Given by Mistake to

5. Now take some time to review the medication exercises you just completed. Use the form below to create an overall analysis of what you have learned. Once again, record each of the medication errors you made, including the type of each error. Then, for each error you made, indicate specifically what you would do differently to prevent this type of error from occurring again.

Medication	Type of Error	Error Prevention Tactic

Submit this form to your instructor if required as a graded assignment, or simply use these exercises to improve your understanding of medication errors and how to reduce them.

Name: _____   Date: _____

The following icons are used throughout this workbook to help you quickly identify particular activities and assignments:

 Indicates a reading assignment—tells you which textbook chapter(s) you should read before starting each lesson

 Indicates a writing activity

 Marks the beginning of an interactive CD-ROM activity—signals you to open or return to your *Virtual Clinical Excursions—General Hospital* CD-ROM

 Indicates additional CD-ROM instructions

 Indicates questions and activities that require you to consult your textbook

 Indicates the approximate time required to complete an exercise

LESSON 1

Priority Setting and Goal Development

 Reading Assignment: Concepts of Health, Illness, Stress, and Health Promotion
(Chapter 2)
Nursing Process and Critical Thinking (Chapter 4)
Assessment, Nursing Diagnosis, and Planning (Chapter 5)
Concepts of Basic Nutrition and Cultural Considerations
(Chapter 26)

Patient: Patricia Newman, Medical-Surgical Floor, Room 406

Objectives:

1. Prioritize nursing diagnoses in order of importance for a patient's well-being.
2. Prioritize tasks appropriately.
3. Develop individualized patient outcomes.

Exercise 1

 CD-ROM Activity—Problems and Nursing Diagnoses

15 minutes

- Sign in to work at Pacific View Regional Hospital on the Medical-Surgical Floor for Period of Care 3. (*Note:* If you are already in the virtual hospital from a previous exercise, click on **Leave the Floor** and then **Restart the Program** to get to the sign-in window.)
- From the Patient List, select Patricia Newman (Room 406).
- Click on **Get Report** for Patricia Newman and take notes as needed.
- Click on **Go to Nurses' Station**.
- Click on **EPR** and then on **Login**.
- Choose **406** as the Patient and **Nutrition** as the Category.

  1. Patricia Newman ate _____% of her breakfast and _____% of her lunch.

 • Click on **Exit EPR**.
- Next, click on **Chart** and then on **406**.
- Click on **Consultations** and read the Dietary Consult.

2. What are the dietary recommendations made by the dietitian?

3. Below, match each NANDA nursing diagnosis with the related problem area.

Problem	Nursing Diagnosis
_____ Discharge	a. Gas exchange, impaired
_____ Fluid/volume electrolyte imbalance	b. Deficient knowledge
_____ Infection	c. Nutrition, less than body requirements
_____ Nutrition	d. Hyperthermia
_____ Respiratory	e. Infection (risk for)
_____ Thermoregulation	f. Fluid volume, risk for imbalanced

4. Match each piece of data below with the nursing diagnosis it supports.

Nursing Diagnosis	Data
_____ Gas exchange, impaired	a. Is eating 30%-40% of meals
_____ Nutrition, less than body requirements	b. Potassium 3.2 mEq/L
_____ Infection (risk for)	c. Temperature 102.5 degrees F
_____ Fluid volume, risk for imbalance	d. Crackles in lower lobes of lungs
_____ Deficient knowledge	e. Is removing nasal oxygen cannula
_____ Hyperthermia	f. White blood cell count 16,000 mm^3

5. The following nursing diagnoses apply to Patricia Newman. Number them in priority order.

Nursing Diagnoses	Order of Priority
_____ Gas exchange, impaired	a. 1
_____ Deficient knowledge	b. 2
_____ Nutrition, less than body requirements	c. 3

6. Write expected outcomes for the three nursing diagnoses listed in the preceding question. (If needed, refer to Chapter 5 in your textbook.)

Exercise 2

 CD-ROM Activity—Priorities Based on Maslow's Hierarchy

 30 minutes

- Sign in to work at Pacific View Regional Hospital on the Medical-Surgical Floor for Period of Care 3. (*Note:* If you are already in the virtual hospital from a previous exercise, click on **Leave the Floor** and then **Restart the Program** to get to the sign-in window.)
- From the Patient List, select Patricia Newman (Room 406).
- Click on **Go to Nurses' Station** and then on **406** at the bottom of the screen.
- Read the **Initial Observations**.
- Click on **Chart** and then on **406**.
- Click on and review the **Nursing Admission**.

   1. a. What is Patricia Newman's height? _____

      b. What is her weight? _____

      c. What is her age? _____

   2. Do you think that Patricia Newman's weight is appropriate for her height and age?

 • Click on the **Laboratory Reports** and note the laboratory values for the various tests.

   3. Which tests results would be the most important to know, considering Patricia Newman's diagnosis of pneumonia?

4. Besides the fact that Patricia Newman is eating only small portions of her meals, what other data have you gathered that support the nursing diagnosis of Nutrition, less than body requirements? Select all that apply.

_____ 5 ft 5 in tall; weight 120 lb

_____ RBCs 4.9

_____ Hematocrit 45

_____ Fatigues easily

_____ Has frequent infections

_____ Needs supplemental oxygen

5. Considering the dietitian's recommendations, Patricia Newman's respiratory status, and her diagnosis of pneumonia, select the action that would be the first priority for her. (*Hint:* Read about pneumonia in your medical-surgical textbook if you need help.)

_____ Explain the importance of keeping the oxygen cannula in place.

_____ Return the oxygen cannula to her nose.

_____ Encourage her to drink 8 oz of water.

_____ Assess what liquids she finds appealing.

_____ Discuss why she should eat more of her meals.

6. Now select the next priority action for Patricia Newman.

_____ Explain the importance of keeping the oxygen cannula in place.

_____ Return the oxygen cannula to her nose.

_____ Encourage her to drink 8 oz of water.

_____ Assess what liquids she finds appealing.

_____ Discuss why she should eat more of her meals.

7. Which of the following would be considered first-level needs for Patricia Newman, according to Maslow's hierarchy? Select all that apply.

_____ Hygiene

_____ Rest and comfort

_____ Psychologic comfort

_____ Affection

_____ Activity

_____ Elimination

_____ Safety

_____ Sexual procreation

_____ Intimacy

_____ Achievement

_____ Learning

2

Critical Thinking and Problem Solving

Reading Assignment: Nursing Process and Critical Thinking (Chapter 4)
Assessment, Nursing Diagnosis, and Planning (Chapter 5)
Assisting with Respiration and Oxygen Delivery (Chapter 28)

Patient: Patricia Newman, Medical-Surgical Floor, Room 406

Objectives:

1. Use critical thinking to gather and analyze data presented in the case study.
2. Use the problem-solving process to decide which assessment data are needed to provide appropriate nursing care for a patient.
3. Use critical thinking in order to organize tasks and set priorities.

Exercise 1

 CD-ROM Activity—Gathering Data

 15 minutes

- Sign in to work at Pacific View Regional Hospital on the Medical-Surgical Floor for Period of Care 1. (*Note:* If you are already in the virtual hospital from a previous exercise, click on **Leave the Floor** and then **Restart the Program** to get to the sign-in window.)
- From the Patient List, select Patricia Newman (Room 406).
- Click on **Get Report** for Patricia Newman and take notes as needed.
- Click on **Go to Nurses' Station**.
- Click on **Chart** and then on **406**. Review the **Physician's Notes** and **Nursing Admission**.

1. Using the change-of-shift report, fill in the following information for Patricia Newman.

   Respiratory status: _____

   Vital signs: BP _____ HR _____ RR _____ T _____ SpO$_2$ _____

   IV: _____

   Priority problem: _____

   Diagnostic tests: _____

2. In the list below, mark with an X those sections of Patricia Newman's patient records you will need to consult at this time to gather necessary data to safely care for her. Select all that apply.

_____ Admissions Records

_____ Operative Reports

_____ Nursing History

_____ Medication Records

_____ History & Physical

_____ Social Services

_____ Physician's Notes

_____ Nurse's Notes

_____ Diagnostic Reports

_____ Kardex

_____ Physician's Orders

→ • Click on **Return to Nurses' Station**.
   • Click on **Kardex** at the top of the screen. Click on **406** and read Patricia Newman's records. (*Remember:* The Kardex provides access to the records of all patients on the floor—not just the patient for whom you are currently caring. Be sure you are looking at the Kardex for the correct room number!)

3. Does Patricia Newman have any allergies that are pertinent to your care for her? (*Hint:* Allergies are listed after the patient problems in the Kardex.)

4. What categories of problems are marked "initiated" on Patricia Newman's Kardex?

5. What are Patricia Newman's diagnoses as listed on the Kardex?

6. Which area is the priority problem for Patricia Newman at this time?

_____ Movement and activity

_____ Circulation

_____ Airway and breathing

_____ Safety

_____ Security

_____ Elimination

Exercise 2

CD-ROM Activity—Priority Assessments and Pulse Oximetry

30 minutes

Read in your textbook about pneumonia and emphysema (COPD).

• Sign in to work at Pacific View Regional Hospital on the Medical-Surgical Floor for Period of Care 1. (*Note:* If you are already in the virtual hospital from a previous exercise, click on **Leave the Floor** and then **Restart the Program** to get to the sign-in window.)
• From the Patient List, select Patricia Newman (Room 406).
• Click on **Go to Nurses' Station**.
• Click on **Chart** and then on **406**.
• Click on **Laboratory Tests**. Read the complete blood count (CBC) report.

1. Patricia Newman's white blood cell count is _____. This is _____ (consistent/inconsistent) with her diagnosis of pneumonia.

2. Considering Patricia Newman's respiratory status and problems, determine assessments that should be performed during your first visit to the patient. From the list below, mark with an X those areas you would assess on your first visit to Patricia Newman.

_____ Vital signs

_____ Verbal complaints

_____ Heart

_____ Lungs

_____ IV

_____ Eyes

_____ Pain level

_____ Skin

_____ Extremities

_____ Abdomen

_____ Neurologic status

➤ • Click on **Return to Nurses' Station**.
   • Now click on **406** at the bottom of your screen to go to Patricia Newman's room.
   • Read the **Initial Observations** and then click on and read the **Clinical Alerts**.

   3. What concerns are highlighted in the Initial Observations and the Clinical Alerts notes?

➤ • Click on **Check Armband** and then on **Take Vital Signs**.

   4. Record Patricia Newman's vital sign measurements below. (*Note:* You will need to enter them in the EPR later.)

   BP _____ T _____ SpO$_2$ _____ HR _____ RR _____ Pain _____

📖 Read about pulse oximetry in your textbook.

   5. How does the pulse oximeter measure oxygen saturation?

   6. Is there a problem with using a fingertip probe for pulse oximetry if the patient is wearing nail polish or artificial nails?

   7. If you didn't want to use Patricia Newman's finger for the pulse oximeter probe, where would you place it?

➤ • Click on **Patient Care** and then on **Chest**.
   • Click on **Respiratory** and note the respiratory assessment data.
   • Click on the **Musculoskeletal** subcategory of the respiratory assessment and note the data that are pertinent regarding respiration.

8. Record the respiratory assessment findings below.

Read about pneumonia in your medical-surgical textbook.

- Click on **Chart** and then on **406**.
- Click on **Laboratory Reports**. Read the CBC report.
- Click on **Diagnostic Reports** and read the x-ray report from Tuesday.

9. Which signs and symptoms of pneumonia does Patricia Newman have? Select all that apply.

_____ Elevated blood pressure

_____ Impaired respiration

_____ Tachycardia

_____ Crackles in lungs

_____ Elevated white blood cell count

_____ Infiltrates on x-ray

_____ Fever

_____ Tachypnea

_____ Diminished aeration

- Click on **Return to Room 406**.
- Click on **EPR** and then on **Login**.
- Choose **406** as the Patient and **Vital Signs** as the Category.
- In the correct column, enter the pain rating and vital signs you recorded in question 4 of this exercise.
- Now choose **Respiratory** from the Category menu. Enter the data you obtained when that system was assessed in question 8.
- Click on the various lines where data are entered to highlight and view the codes used for that part of the system. (*Hint:* The code meanings are listed to the right of the data columns.)

10. What differences did you find between what you just charted and what was charted for these systems on Wednesday at 0300?

Exercise 3

 CD-ROM Activity—Problem Solving and Prioritizing

 30 minutes

- Sign in to work at Pacific View Regional Hospital on the Medical-Surgical Floor for Period of Care 1. (*Note:* If you are already in the virtual hospital from a previous exercise, click on **Leave the Floor** and then **Restart the Program** to get to the sign-in window.)
- From the Patient List, select **Patricia Newman** (Room 406).
- Click on **Go to Nurses' Station**.

1. Which area is the priority problem for Patricia Newman at this time?

_____ Movement and activity

_____ Circulation

_____ Airway and oxygenation

_____ Safety

_____ Security

- Click on **Chart** and then on **406**.
- Click on **History and Physical** and read the records.

2. Patricia Newman has been hospitalized for pneumonia multiple times in the past 2 years. What do you think are contributing factors for this problem?

3. You will be expected to do discharge teaching for Patricia Newman during her hospital stay. How would you approach the topic of recurrent pneumonia? Review the actions listed below and number them in the order in which you would use them.

Action	Order of Priority
_____ Give the patient smoking cessation literature to read.	a. 1
	b. 2
_____ Find out how she feels about the repeated hospitalizations.	c. 3
_____ Ask whether she has ever tried to quit smoking.	d. 4
_____ Explain how smoking predisposes her to lung infection.	e. 5
_____ Provide a list of community resources for quitting smoking.	

4. What actions can you teach Patricia Newman to do at home that will help to keep her lungs clear? (*Hint:* Review pneumonia and nursing interventions in your medical-surgical textbook.)

Exercise 4

 CD-ROM Activity—Interventions to Meet Expected Outcomes

 15 minutes

- Sign in to work at Pacific View Regional Hospital on the Medical-Surgical Floor for Period of Care 1. (*Note:* If you are already in the virtual hospital from a previous exercise, click on **Leave the Floor** and then **Restart the Program** to get to the sign-in window.)
- From the Patient List, select Patricia Newman (Room 406).
- Click on **Go to Nurses' Station**.
- Click on **MAR** and then on tab **406** to view Patricia Newman's MAR. Scroll down to the second page of the MAR.

1. Atenolol has been ordered to manage Patricia Newman's hypertension. What impact will this medication have on her cardiac output and heart rate? (*Hint:* Refer to the Drug Guide.)

2. Atenolol will increase the myocardial oxygen demand.
   a. True
   b. False

3. When preparing to administer atenolol, which of the following nursing actions is indicated? Select all that apply.

   _____ Measure the patient's temperature.

   _____ Measure the apical pulse.

   _____ Measure the blood pressure.

   _____ Assess respirations.

   _____ Check renal function and liver function laboratory results.

   _____ Auscultate lung fields.

Communication and the Nurse-Patient Relationship

 Reading Assignment: Documentation of Nursing Care (Chapter 7)
Communication and the Nurse-Patient Relationship (Chapter 8)

Patients: Harry George, Medical-Surgical Floor, Room 401
Clarence Hughes, Medical-Surgical Floor, Room 404
William Jefferson, Skilled Nursing Unit, Room 501

Objectives:

1. List the factors that influence the way a person communicates.
2. Differentiate effective communication techniques from those that block communication.
3. Identify effective techniques to gather information from patients.
4. Document patient care appropriately.

Exercise 1

 CD-ROM Activity—Communication Skills

30 minutes

- Sign in to work at Pacific View Regional Hospital on the Medical-Surgical Floor for Period of Care 1. (*Note:* If you are already in the virtual hospital from a previous exercise, click on **Leave the Floor** and then **Restart the Program** to get to the sign-in window.)
- From the Patient List, select Harry George (Room 401).
- Click on **Get Report**.
- Read the report and note any data indicating a possible problem.
- Click on **Go to Nurses' Station** and then on **401** to visit the patient's room.
- Click on **Patient Care** and then on **Nurse-Client Interactions**.
- Select and view the video titled **0735: Symptom Management**. (*Note:* Check the virtual clock to see whether enough time has elapsed. You can use the fast-forward feature to advance the time by 2-minute intervals if the video is not yet available. Then click again on **Patient Care** and **Nurse-Client Interactions** to refresh the screen.)

1. Review Harry George's nonverbal behavior during the exchange with the sitter. Describe what you observe for each of the elements listed below.

Personal appearance

Facial expression

Eye contact

2. Review the sitter's response to Harry George's complaints. Which of the following communication techniques does he attempt to employ?
   a. Restating
   b. Clarifying
   c. Touch
   d. Summarizing

3. During the interaction between Harry George and the sitter, Harry George's nonverbal behavior is consistent with his spoken comments.
   a. True
   b. False

4. The term _____ is used to describe an inconsistency between verbal and nonverbal behaviors.

5. During the interaction, the nurse approaches Harry George and inquires about his level of pain and the effectiveness of the analgesics given. Describe the nurse's entry into the patient's personal space. Was it appropriate?

6. As she begins the conversation with Harry George, the nurse asks him about the effective-

   ness of his pain medication. The nurse phrases this as a(n) _____-ended question.

7. After Harry George expressed his belief that alcohol would make him feel better, the nurse provided him with education related to the dangers of his behavior. Was this the appropriate response by the nurse? What factors should the nurse pay close attention to when providing such information?

8. Review the nurse's interaction with Harry George. Do you have any concerns about the manner in which the nurse interacted with him?

9. Compare and contrast the report from the Initial Observations at 0730 and Harry George's demeanor during the 0735 Nurse-Client Interaction.

10. To demonstrate empathy for Harry George, which of the following would be appropriate? Select all that apply.

_____ Reflection of the patient's expressed thoughts

_____ Focus on the patient's feelings

_____ Very close physical proximity to the patient

_____ A warm tone of voice

_____ Suggestions on how to best solve the patient's problems

_____ A nonjudgmental attitude

- Click on **Patient Care** and then on **Nurse-Client Interactions**.
- Select and view the video titled **0755: Disease Management**. (*Note:* Check the virtual clock to see whether enough time has elapsed. You can use the fast-forward feature to advance the time by 2-minute intervals if the video is not yet available. Then click again on **Patient Care** and **Nurse-Client Interactions** to refresh the screen.)

11. In response to Harry George's complaints of pain, which of the following communication techniques is being employed by the sitter?
a. Empathy
b. Restatement
c. Distraction
d. Touch

12. The sitter's provision of information to Harry George is appropriate given his professional status.
a. True
b. False

- Click on **Patient Care** and then on **Nurse-Client Interactions**.
- Select and view the video titled **0810: The Patient in Pain**. (*Note:* Check the virtual clock to see whether enough time has elapsed. You can use the fast-forward feature to advance the time by 2-minute intervals if the video is not yet available. Then click again on **Patient Care** and **Nurse-Client Interactions** to refresh the screen.)

13. Compare the nurse's demeanor in this interaction with that in the earlier (0735) video. Which do you think is more appropriate?

Exercise 2

 CD-ROM Activity—Communication Techniques

 30 minutes

* Sign in to work at Pacific View Regional Hospital on the Skilled Nursing Floor for Period of Care 1. (*Note:* If you are already in the virtual hospital from a previous exercise, click on **Leave the Floor** and then **Restart the Program** to get to the sign-in window.)
* From the Patient List, select William Jefferson (Room 501).
* Click on **Get Report** and read the **Clinical Report**.
* Click on **Go to Nurses' Station**.
* Click on **Chart** and then on **501**.
* Click on and review the **History and Physical**.
* Click on **Return to Nurses' Station** and then on **501** to go to the patient's room.
* Read the **Initial Observations**.

1. What psychosocial issues could affect the nurse's communication with William Jefferson? How might these behaviors affect the interaction?

2. What physiologic and environmental issues being experienced by William Jefferson may affect the nurse-patient interaction?

3. Which of the following interventions will assist the nurse in establishing a positive rapport when communicating with William Jefferson? Select all that apply.

    _____   Assist the patient to the dining room to promote feelings of socialization.

    _____   Face him during interactions.

    _____   Avoid analgesic administration to reduce drowsiness during interactions.

    _____   Provide adequate lighting during interactions.

    _____   Use touch as culturally appropriate.

4. When the nurse is caring for William Jefferson, which of the following variables will have the most influence on communication?
    a. His age and race
    b. His culture and social position
    c. Scheduled agenda for the day
    d. Race of the care provider
    e. Disorientation and confusion

➤ • Click on **Patient Care** and then on **Nurse-Client Interactions**.
• Select and view the video titled **0730: Intervention—Patient Safety**. (*Note:* Check the virtual clock to see whether enough time has elapsed. You can use the fast-forward feature to advance the time by 2-minute intervals if the video is not yet available. Then click again on **Patient Care** and **Nurse-Client Interactions** to refresh the screen.)

5. Review and critique the nurse's interaction with William Jefferson. What behaviors indicate that the nurse is attempting to establish a rapport with him?

6. Which of the following is the primary concern for the nurse during the interaction?

    _____   The safety of the patient

    _____   The patient's disorientation

    _____   Locating the patient's family members

    _____   The patient's ability to tolerate ambulation

➤ • Click on **Patient Care** and then on **Nurse-Client Interactions**.
• Select and view the video titled **0740: The Confused Patient**. (*Note:* Check the virtual clock to see whether enough time has elapsed. You can use the fast-forward feature to advance the time by 2-minute intervals if the video is not yet available. Then click again on **Patient Care** and **Nurse-Client Interactions** to refresh the screen.)

7. During the interaction, what communication techniques are used by the nurse?

8. The nurse's initial attempts to touch William Jefferson are rebuffed. Are repeated attempts appropriate?

9. Review William Jefferson's appearance and behaviors during the exchange. List your findings for each area below.

Personal appearance

Facial expression

Eye contact

→ • Click on **Patient Care** and then on **Nurse-Client Interactions**.
   • Select and view the video titled **0745: Intervention—Redirection**. (*Note:* Check the virtual clock to see whether enough time has elapsed. You can use the fast-forward feature to advance the time by 2-minute intervals if the video is not yet available. Then click again on **Patient Care** and **Nurse-Client Interactions** to refresh the screen.)

10. What is the primary underlying purpose of the communication technique being demonstrated by the nurse during the interaction?
    a. Distraction
    b. Assessment of patient's cognition
    c. Assessment of patient's personal interests
    d. Evaluation of patient's needs

11. How does William Jefferson's demeanor and interaction with the nurse in this exchange differ from the previous interaction?

Exercise 3

 CD-ROM Activity—Communication and Empathy

 45 minutes

- Sign in to work at Pacific View Regional Hospital on the Medical-Surgical Floor for Period of Care 1. (*Note:* If you are already in the virtual hospital from a previous exercise, click on **Leave the Floor** and then **Restart the Program** to get to the sign-in window.)
- From the Patient List, select Clarence Hughes (Room 404).
- Click on **Get Report**.
- Read the report and note any data indicating a possible problem.
- Click on **Go to Nurses' Station** and then on **404** to visit the patient's room.
- Click on **Patient Care** and then on **Nurse-Client Interactions**.
- Select and view the video titled **0730: Assessment/Perception of Care**. (*Note:* Check the virtual clock to see whether enough time has elapsed. You can use the fast-forward feature to advance the time by 2-minute intervals if the video is not yet available. Then click again on **Patient Care** and **Nurse-Client Interactions** to refresh the screen.)

1. What nonverbal actions and/or signs did you observe while watching Clarence Hughes?

2. Do the nonverbal messages agree with what Clarence Hughes is saying to the nurse?

3. Do you think it is appropriate for the nurse to ask to do the assessment before giving Clarence Hughes the pain medication he is requesting? Why or why not?

 • Click on **Patient Care** and then on **Nurse-Client Interactions**.
- Select and view the video titled **0735: Empathy**. (*Note:* Check the virtual clock to see whether enough time has elapsed. You can use the fast-forward feature to advance the time by 2-minute intervals if the video is not yet available. Then click again on **Patient Care** and **Nurse-Client Interactions** to refresh the screen.)

4. Was the nurse's first question to Clarence Hughes therapeutic or nontherapeutic? What type of technique did the nurse use by asking this question?

Read about knee arthroplasty and continuous passive motion (CPM) in your textbook.

5. Is the nurse showing empathy for Clarence Hughes' pain of 8/10 when she says she will put the CPM back on after giving him his pain medication?

6. Which of the following are used when empathy is present? Select all that apply.

_____ Reflection of the person's expressed thought

_____ Focus on the person's feelings

_____ Very close physical proximity

_____ Warm tone of voice

_____ Suggestions on how to solve the problem

_____ A nonjudgmental attitude

• Still in Clarence Hughes' room, click on **Initial Observations** and read the note.
• Now click on **Clinical Alerts** and read the note.
• Click on **Take Vital Signs**.

7. Record Clarence Hughes' vital signs below.

BP _____ T _____ SpO$_2$ _____ HR _____ RR _____ Pain _____

• Click on **Patient Care** and then on **Physical Assessment**.
• Click on **Lower Extremities** and obtain a focused assessment on Clarence Hughes by clicking on each of the subcategories in green boxes. (*Note:* Jot down pertinent findings so that you will be able to document the assessment later.)

8. Using your assessment data and the information from the video interactions, write a SOAP note below regarding Clarence Hughes' pain and surgical site just as you would for the patient's chart.

S

O

A

P

→ • Click on **EPR** in the upper right area of the screen. Click on **Login**.
   • Select **404** as the Patient and **Vital Signs** as the Category.
   • In the correct column, enter the vital signs and pain assessment data you obtained during this exercise. Highlight each pertinent line to view the codes and meanings available to you.
   • Click on **Exit EPR** and then on **Chart**. Click on **404** and select **Nurse's Notes**.
   • Read the note relevant to the 0730 Nurse-Client Interaction you observed earlier.

9. What type of documentation did the nurse use to write this nurse's note?

_____ POMR

_____ DAR

_____ PIE

_____ Focus charting

_____ Narrative charting

_____ Charting by exception

10. Is the information obtained from the patient about his pain subjective or objective data?

Documentation of Nursing Care

 Reading Assignment: Documentation of Nursing Care (Chapter 7)

Patients: Harry George, Medical-Surgical Floor, Room 401
Clarence Hughes, Medical-Surgical Floor, Room 404

Objectives:

1. Document patient care in electronic patient records.
2. Identify data that should be documented in the nurse's notes.
3. Correctly document in the nurse's notes.
4. List data that should be included when documenting a change in condition.

Exercise 1

CD-ROM Activity—Exploring Documentation

30 minutes

- Sign in to work at Pacific View Regional Hospital on the Medical-Surgical Floor for Period of Care 2. (*Note:* If you are already in the virtual hospital from a previous exercise, click on **Leave the Floor** and then **Restart the Program** to get to the sign-in window.)
- From the Patient List, select Clarence Hughes (Room 404).
- Click on **Get Report** and review.
- Click on **Go to Nurses' Station** and then on **404**.
- Inside the patient's room, click on **Take Vital Signs**.

1. Record Clarence Hughes' current vital signs below.

   BP _____ SpO$_2$ _____ T _____ HR _____ RR _____ Pain _____

 • Read the **Initial Observations**.
- Click on **Clinical Alerts** and read the note.
- Click on **Patient Care** and then on **Nurse-Client Interactions**.
- Select and view the video titled **1115: Interventions—Airway**. (*Note:* Check the virtual clock to see whether enough time has elapsed. You can use the fast-forward feature to

advance the time by 2-minute intervals if the video is not yet available. Then click again on **Patient Care** and **Nurse-Client Interactions** to refresh the screen.)

- Now click on **Patient Care** and then **Physical Assessment**.
- Click on **Chest** and then on each subcategory for the chest assessment, noting any abnormal data.
- Click on **EPR** and then on **Login**. Select **404** as the Patient and **Vital Signs** as the Category.
- In the correct column, enter the vital sign data you obtained in question 1.
- Now select **Respiratory** from the Category menu. Enter the data you obtained during that portion of the chest assessment. Highlight each line to see the codes and meanings you may use for that specific item.
- Next, choose **Cardiovascular** and enter that assessment data.
- Finally, select **Psychosocial** and enter the data regarding Clarence Hughes' anxiety.
- Return to the **Vital Signs** category.

2. Which vital sign measurements have changed considerably since they were last taken? Select all that apply.

_____   Blood pressure

_____   Temperature

_____   Heart rate

_____   SpO$_2$

_____   Respiratory rate

3. What nonverbal communication did you observe in the video interaction that indicated Clarence Hughes is in distress?

4. Using a focus charting format, write a nurse's note regarding the change in Clarence Hughes' condition. (*Hint:* See page 91 in your textbook.)

D

A

R

• Before leaving the EPR, familiarize yourself with the various available charting sections of this electronic format by choosing each category in turn and reviewing the data lines available for that area.

- Now click on **Exit EPR** and then on **Chart**. Select **404** and click on **Nurse's Notes**.
- Compare the nurse's note in the chart with the note you wrote for question 4.

5. Did you leave anything important out of the nurse's note you wrote for question 4?

Exercise 2

 CD-ROM Activity—Documentation Practice

 45 minutes

- Sign in to work at Pacific View Regional Hospital on the Medical-Surgical Floor for Period of Care 1. (*Note:* If you are already in the virtual hospital from a previous exercise, click on **Leave the Floor** and then **Restart the Program** to get to the sign-in window.)
- From the Patient List, select Harry George (Room 401).
- Click on **Get Report** and read the report.
- Click on **Go to Nurses' Station** and then on **401** to go to Harry George's room.
- Read the **Initial Observations**.
- Click on **Clinical Alerts** to determine whether there is an immediate nursing need.
- Click on **Take Vital Signs**.

1. What are Harry George's current vital signs?

   BP __132/96__ SpO$_2$ __90__ T __100.8__ HR __101__ RR __18__ Pain __6__

 • Begin a brief assessment on Harry George by clicking on **Patient Care** and then on **Physical Assessment**.

- Then click on **Head & Neck** (from the column of yellow boxes) and then on **Mental Status** from the subcategories (green boxes).

2. What is Harry George's current mental status?

   A+O x 4
   Speech appropriate
   Intermittent agitation and combativeness c̄ expressed frustration of high pain level and limited mobility.

 • Click on **Lower Extremities** and then on each of the available subcategories.

- Make note of any pertinent findings for later entry in the EPR or for writing a nurse's note.

3. What do your findings from the assessment of Harry George's lower extremities reveal?

skin warm/dry erythematous over anterior tibial surface intact s̄ lesion, left leg erythematedematous from toe to mid calf. open lesion 2-3cm in size on Ⓛ ankle draining serous fluid. impaired range of motion, sensation and movement in Ⓛ leg. In Ⓡ leg Full ROM sensation and movement. cap. refill sluggish at 4 seconds. Femoral and popiteal pulse 2+ bl laterally. Posterior tibialis and dorsalis pedis pulsed diminished 1+ doppler. pedal pulse 2+ on right. Intermittant mild tremors reflexes intact sensation and strength in Ⓛ leg unpaired c̄ pain response +. touch sensation and strength in Ⓡ leg s̄ deficits.

→ • Click on **EPR** in the right corner of the screen and then click **Login**.

• Select **401** as the Patient and **Vital Signs** as the Category.

• Locate the Wed 0730 time column. Record your vital signs findings from question 1.

• Now choose **Cardiovascular** from the Category menu and enter the data you obtained from the vascular assessment of the lower extremities.

• Next, select **Neurologic** and enter the data you obtained regarding Harry George's mental status.

• Then choose **Musculoskeletal** and enter the data you obtained when you assessed the lower extremities.

• Now select **Integumentary** and enter the appropriate code for the assessment of the lower extremities.

• Finally, select **Wounds and Drains** and enter the codes for the assessment of Harry George's leg wound.

4. Now write a nurse's note for the remaining assessment data that you could not record in the EPR. Use source-oriented or narrative charting. (*Hint:* See pages 87-88 in your textbook.)

A+O x4. Aggitated and combativeness c̄ frustration of pain. vitals obtain BP 130/90, S02 90, resp 18, HR/puls 101 temp 100.8 pain at 6. Ⓡ leg no appeared deficet. Ⓛ leg swollen, lesion 2-3cm on toe to mid calf. impaired ability in Ⓛ leg. call light within reach.

→ • Click on **Exit EPR**.

• Click on **Chart** and then **401**.

• Click on the **Physician's Orders**. Find the order for pain medication.

5. The medication order written for Harry George's pain is

ceftazidmine 2 g IV every 8 hours.

→ • Click on **Return to Room 401** and then on **MAR**. Select tab **401** and search for the pain medication you found in the physician's order.

6. Harry George received the new pain medication at *0800, 1600 2400*

• Click on **Return to Room 401**.
   • Click on **Chart** and then **401**.
   • Click on the **Nurse's Notes** and read the note for the beginning of this shift.

7. What does the nurse's note say about Harry George's pain level and administration of pain medication?

10/10 and Hydromorphone 2 mg given IV, within 30 min, pain rating went down.

Exercise 3

 CD-ROM Activity—Other Charting Formats

 30 minutes

• Sign in to work at Pacific View Regional Hospital on the Medical-Surgical Floor for Period of Care 1. (*Note:* If you are already in the virtual hospital from a previous exercise, click on **Leave the Floor** and then **Restart the Program** to get to the sign-in window.)
• From the Patient List, select Harry George (Room 401).
• Click on **Go to Nurses' Station**.

1. Data obtained from the patient verbally are called subjective data. Data obtained by hands-on physical assessment or through the nurse's own senses are objective data. Match each piece of data below with its correct data type.

Data	Data Type
S "My pain is at 8/10."	a. Subjective
O Left lower leg erythematous from toes to mid-calf.	b. Objective
S "It hurts to move my foot."	
O Serous drainage from wound.	
O Temperature 100.2 degrees F.	
S "Bring me my bottle and a cigarette."	

2. Match each piece of assessment data listed below with the location in the patient record where it should be documented.

Data Obtained

_c_ Open lesion 2-3 cm on left ankle

_c_ Right pedal pulse 2+

_a_ Pain at 6/10

_a_ Skin erythematous from toes to mid-calf of left leg

_b_ Impaired ROM in left leg

_a_ Asking for alcohol and cigarettes

_g_ Alert and oriented to person, place, and situation

_c_ Hydromorphone 2 mg IV given at 0715

Where to Document Data

a. Chart only

b. EPR only

c. Chart and EPR

3. The charting by exception format assumes that _____, unless documented to the contrary. (*Hint:* See page 91 in your textbook.)
   a. the body system was assessed
   b. data obtained are irrelevant
   c. all standards and protocols were followed
   d. a full physical assessment has been performed

4. Which of the following are true of the charting guidelines for correct, legally accurate documentation? Select all that apply.

   _____ Use only agency-accepted symbols and abbreviations in documentation.

   ✓ Visitors should be mentioned by name.

   ✓ Physician visits should be documented.

   _____ Start each sentence with a capital letter and end with a period.

   _____ Use complete sentences when documenting in the nurse's notes.

   _____ When the patient is the subject of the sentence, leave "patient" out of the sentence.

   _____ Do not duplicate the charting of an item on a flow sheet in the nurse's notes.

   ✓ Chart only what you have performed or observed.

   _____ Pencil may be used on a flow sheet.

   ✓ Entries must not be erased or covered with any type of correction fluid.

- Click on **401** to go to the patient's room.
- Click on **Patient Care** and then on **Nurse-Client Interactions**.
- Select and view the video titled **0810: The Patient in Pain**. (*Note:* Check the virtual clock to see whether enough time has elapsed. You can use the fast-forward feature to advance the time by 2-minute intervals if the video is not yet available. Then click again on **Patient Care** and **Nurse-Client Interactions** to refresh the screen.)

5. Write a SOAP note regarding the interaction you just observed. (*Hint:* Review the SOAP format on page 89 of your textbook.)

S

O

A

P

6. PIE charting is another style of charting. Document the nurse-client interaction you observed using the PIE format.

P

I

E

LESSON 5

Patient Teaching

 Reading Assignment: Patient Teaching for Health Promotion (Chapter 9)

Patients: Piya Jordan, Medical-Surgical Floor, Room 403
Clarence Hughes, Medical-Surgical Floor, Room 404
Patricia Newman, Medical-Surgical Floor, Room 406

Objectives:

1. Identify areas of knowledge deficit for patients.
2. Recognize factors that may affect learning for individual patients.
3. Determine the best methods for teaching specific content.
4. Devise individualized teaching plans.

Exercise 1

 CD-ROM Activity—Assessing Learning Needs

 30 minutes

Review the factors that affect learning on pages 114-115 of your textbook.

- Sign in to work at Pacific View Regional Hospital on the Medical-Surgical Floor for Period of Care 3. (*Note:* If you are already in the virtual hospital from a previous exercise, click on **Leave the Floor** and then **Restart the Program** to get to the sign-in window.)
- From the Patient List, select Patricia Newman (Room 406).
- Click on **Go to Nurses' Station**.
- Click on **Chart** and then on **406**.
- Click on the **Nursing Admission**.

1. What factors mentioned in the chart do you think may interfere with learning for Patricia Newman at this time? Select all that apply.

_____ Pain

_____ Fatigue

_____ Fever

_____ Anxiety

_____ Decreased oxygenation

_____ Nausea

_____ Sedation

_____ Visitor

Review the Modes of Learning and Factors Affecting Learning in your textbook.

2. Based on your review of the Nursing Admission assessment, you determine that Patricia

   Newman most likely learns best by _____ _____. This means that

   she is primarily a(n) _____ (auditory/visual/kinesthetic) learner.

3. What methods would you use in carrying out Patricia Newman's teaching plan?

4. Assess the following factors that might affect Patricia Newman's learning.

Primary language

Memory

Vision

Barriers to learning

Secondary language

Hearing

Literacy level

5. Did you discover any cultural factors that might affect Patricia Newman's willingness to learn or the way you should plan teaching for her?

6. A nursing diagnosis related to Patricia Newman's learning needs would be _____

_____.

→ • Click on **Return to Nurses' Station** and then on **406**.
   • Inside the patient's room, click on **Patient Care** and then on **Nurse-Client Interactions**.
   • Select and view the video titled **1500: Discharge Planning**. (*Note:* Check the virtual clock to see whether enough time has elapsed. You can use the fast-forward feature to advance the time by 2-minute intervals if the video is not yet available. Then click again on **Patient Care** and **Nurse-Client Interactions** to refresh the screen.)
   • After viewing the video, click on **Chart** and then on **406**. Select the **Patient Education** tab and read the education plan.

7. What seems to be missing from this plan, considering the video interaction you just viewed?

8. List eight areas of education that need to be addressed for Patricia Newman.

9. Consider the following areas of teaching in regard to Patricia Newman's care: diet management, disease condition, medication compliance, smoking cessation, activity, and self-care.

   a. Which of these teaching areas would be the first priority?

   b. Which would be the second priority?

10. Which of the following resources do you think would be helpful for your teaching plan? Select all that apply.

_____ Dietitian's help in planning meals

_____ Pictures of each medication

_____ Video on correct use of MDI

_____ Information and printed materials on community smoking cessation programs

_____ Drug inserts on her medications

_____ A chart for progress with progressive ambulation

_____ Booklet on emphysema and its treatment

_____ Statistics on death from smoking

_____ Chart and schedule for medication administration

_____ Demonstration of effective coughing

_____ Examples of high-protein snacks

_____ Pamphlet on proper MDI use

Exercise 2

CD-ROM Activity—Teaching Self-Injection

⏱ 30 minutes

- Sign in to work at Pacific View Regional Hospital on the Medical-Surgical Floor for Period of Care 2. (*Note:* If you are already in the virtual hospital from a previous exercise, click on **Leave the Floor** and then **Restart the Program** to get to the sign-in window.)
- From the Patient List, select Clarence Hughes (Room 404).
- Click on **Chart** and then on **404**. Click on the tab for **Nursing Admission** and read the assessment, noting factors that are pertinent to Clarence Hughes' learning.

1. Clarence Hughes states that he learns best by what methods?

2. How does Clarence Hughes describe his short- and long-term memory?

3. What problem does he indicate he has that will have an impact on teaching-learning sessions?

4. What would you do to help with this problem?

5. What other factor (specific to Clarence Hughes) needs to be considered when planning his teaching-learning sessions?

6. Once his pain is within tolerable limits, what teaching needs are important for Clarence Hughes?

7. Consider the events that have been taking place during Clarence Hughes' hospitalization. Identify the two greatest educational needs for him at this time.

_____ Prevention of osteoporosis

_____ Pain management

_____ Management/prevention of constipation

_____ Eating a balanced diet

8. Clarence Hughes will need to continue his enoxaparin injections at home. Use the format below to devise a teaching plan for him.

Medication Teaching Plan

Topic	Behavioral Objective	Evaluation Method

Exercise 3

 CD-ROM Activity—Factors Affecting Learning

15 minutes

- Sign in to work at Pacific View Regional Hospital on the Medical-Surgical Floor for Period of Care 1. (*Note:* If you are already in the virtual hospital from a previous exercise, click on **Leave the Floor** and then **Restart the Program** to get to the sign-in window.)
- From the Patient List, select Piya Jordan (Room 403).
- Click on **Go to Nurses' Station**.
- Click on **Chart** and then on **403**.
- Review the **Laboratory Reports** and the **Nursing Admission**.
- Click on **Physician's Notes** and review the notes.

1. Which of the following factors might interfere with Piya Jordan's ability to learn at the present time? Select all that apply.

_____ Fatigue

_____ Lack of family support

_____ NPO status

_____ Electrolyte imbalance

_____ Poor hearing

_____ Pain

_____ Nausea

_____ Tubes and drains

_____ Anemia

_____ Fear

_____ Confusion

_____ Inadequate oxygenation

2. Piya Jordan's best methods of learning are _____ and

_____.

3. What level of education does Piya Jordan have?

4. Piya Jordan was formerly employed as a _____ _____.

5. How might her former occupation be useful now?

6. If Piya Jordan's tumor turns out to be adenocarcinoma of the colon, she will need chemotherapy. Can you count on her husband to support her during treatment?

7. What other support might be available to Piya Jordan?

8. What cultural factors should be taken into consideration when formulating a teaching plan for Piya Jordan?

LESSON 6

Nursing Care of the Elderly: Common Physical Care Issues

Reading Assignment: Promoting Healthy Adaptation to Aging (Chapter 13)
Lifting, Moving, and Positioning Patients (Chapter 18)
Common Physical Care Problems of the Elderly (Chapter 40)
Common Psychocsocial Care Problems of the Elderly
(Chapter 41)

Patients: William Jefferson, Skilled Nursing Floor, Room 501
Kathryn Doyle, Skilled Nursing Floor, Room 503

Objectives:

1. Identify interventions to assist the confused elderly patient.
2. Discuss age-related physiologic changes that predispose older adults to problems.
3. Examine factors related to polypharmacy.
4. Incorporate fall prevention measures into daily care.

Exercise 1

 CD-ROM Activity—The Patient with Dementia

 30 minutes

- Sign in to work at Pacific View Regional Hospital on the Skilled Nursing Floor for Period of Care 1. (*Note:* If you are already in the virtual hospital from a previous exercise, click on **Leave the Floor** and then **Restart the Program** to get to the sign-in window.)
- From the Patient List, select William Jefferson (Room 501).
- Click on **Get Report** and review. Then click on **Go to Nurses' Station**.
- Click on **501** to visit William Jefferson. Read the **Initial Observations**.
- Click on **Chart** and then on **501**. Open the **History and Physical** and review.

1. What significant illnesses/disorders are discussed in William Jefferson's History and Physical?

2. According to the History and Physical, William Jefferson was diagnosed with Alzheimer's

   disease _____ years ago.

3. What stage of Alzheimer's disease is William Jefferson in?

4. Which of the following manifestations is associated with the late stage of Alzheimer's disease?
   a. Wandering
   b. Intermittent confusion
   c. Weight loss
   d. Incontinence

5. Mental declines are a normal part of the aging process.
   a. True
   b. False

6. Anxiety can result in an elder person displaying decreases in cognition.
   a. True
   b. False

→ • Click on **Return to Room 501** and then click on **Patient Care**.
   • Click on **Nurse-Client Interactions**.
   • Select and view the video titled **0730: Intervention—Patient Safety**.
   • Then select and watch the video titled **0740: The Confused Patient**. (*Note:* Check the virtual clock to see whether enough time has elapsed. You can use the fast-forward feature to advance the time by 2-minute intervals if the video is not yet available. Then click again on **Patient Care** and **Nurse-Client Interactions** to refresh the screen.)

7. What is the situation in the first (0730) interaction?

8. How does the second (0740) interaction demonstrate William Jefferson's confusion? What technique does the nurse use to handle the situation?

9. Given William Jefferson's confusion and attempts to ambulate on his own, restraints are indicated.
   a. True
   b. False

10. William Jefferson is concerned about the location of his dog. Base on your understanding, what impact do animals have on the confused elder? Select all that apply.

_____ Caring for animals is a source of stress for the confused elder.

_____ Animals provide a source of tactile stimulation.

_____ Animal care provides a source of industry/purpose for the elder.

_____ Animals can fill the void of loneliness.

⟶ • Click on **Chart** and then on **501**. Select the **Nursing Admission** and read more about William Jefferson.

11. What social interaction does William Jefferson have when outside of the hospital?

12. What impact does social interaction have on the elder who is experiencing confusion?

Exercise 2

 CD-ROM Activity—Physical Problems of the Elderly

 45 minutes

Recall that William Jefferson was admitted with a urinary tract infection and sepsis. His diabetes and blood pressure were not controlled at the time of admission.

• Sign in to work at Pacific View Regional Hospital on the Skilled Nursing Floor for Period of Care 1. (*Note:* If you are already in the virtual hospital from a previous exercise, click on **Leave the Floor** and then **Restart the Program** to get to the sign-in window.)
• From the Patient List, select William Jefferson (Room 501).
• Click on **Get Report** and read the report.
• Click on **Go to Nurses' Station**.

1. How do decreased bladder tone and incomplete emptying predispose older adults to urinary tract infection?

2. What physiologic changes related to aging in males can contribute to the occurrence of the problems mentioned in question 1?

 3. How does benign prostatic hypertrophy add to the problem of decreased bladder tone? (*Hint:* Read in your medical-surgical textbook about this disorder.)

4. Which of the following would you include in your teaching plan for William Jefferson and his wife in order to prevent recurrent cystitis? Select all that apply.

_____ Increase fluid intake to 1800 mL per day

_____ Empty the bladder every 2 hours

_____ Drink cranberry juice daily

_____ Take a Vitamin B_1 supplement

_____ Increase fluid intake to 2500-3000 mL per day

_____ Empty the bladder every hour

_____ Avoid most citrus fruits and juice

_____ Take a vitamin C supplement

William Jefferson developed sepsis, which in this case was a systemic inflammatory response to the infection. Sepsis can be fatal. It is important that the patient and his wife receive adequate teaching about prevention of future urinary tract infections. William Jefferson also has hypertension, diabetes, and osteoarthritis. Several medications have been prescribed for his various conditions.

→ • Click on **MAR** and select tab **501** for William Jefferson's records.

5. Below, list the regularly scheduled medication orders written for William Jefferson. For each medication, provide the action and explain why the patient is receiving it.

Medication Order	Action	Reason for Receiving

6. Why is taking multiple medications such a problem for an elderly person?

7. The use of nonprescription drugs such as _____ or

_____ can alter drug elimination from the body.

→ • Click on **Return to Nurses' Station**. Now click on **Medication Room** and begin to prepare William Jefferson's 0800 medications.
• Click on **Unit Dosage** or on the unit dosage cart. Select drawer **501** to see a list of the medications ordered for William Jefferson.
• Click on one of the drugs you need to administer at 0800.
• Compare the unit dosage label with the MAR order; then click **Put Medication on Tray**.
• Repeat the previous two steps for each 0800 medication.
• Now perform your second check by clicking on **Review Your Medications** and following the Five Rights.

- After verifying your medications, click on **Return to Medication Room**, then on **Close Drawer**, and then on **View Medication Room**.
- Click on **Preparation** in the upper left corner of your screen.
- Prepare each medication by clicking on the drug name and supplying any information requested by the Preparation Wizard.
- When all medications are properly prepared and verified, click on **Finish** and then on **Return to Medication Room**.
- Now click on **501**, **Patient Care**, and **Medication Administration**.
- Administer all of William Jefferson's 0800 medications using the Five Rights and following the prompts of the Administration Wizard.
- When finished, click on **Leave the Floor** and then on **Look at Your Preceptor's Evaluation**. Finally, select **Medication Scorecard** to see how you did.

8. Did you make any errors? If so, what were they? What would you do differently next time?

Exercise 3

 CD-ROM Activity—Fall Prevention

 15 minutes

- Sign in to work at Pacific View Regional Hospital on the Skilled Nursing Floor for Period of Care 1. (*Note:* If you are already in the virtual hospital from a previous exercise, click on **Leave the Floor** and then **Restart the Program** to get to the sign-in window.)
- From the Patient List, select Kathryn Doyle (Room 503).
- Click on **Get Report** and read the report.
- Click on **Go to Nurses' Station**.
- Now click on **Chart** and then on **503**. Click on the tab for **History and Physical**.

Kathryn Doyle is in the Skilled Nursing Unit for rehabilitation after the hip surgery.

1. What medical conditions are listed in Kathryn Doyle's History and Physical?

 • Click on **Return to Nurses' Station** and then on **503**.
- Click on **Clinical Alerts** and review the note.
- Click on **Patient Care** and then on **Nurse-Client Interactions**.
- Select and view the video titled **0730: Assessment—Biopsychosocial**. (*Note:* Check the virtual clock to see whether enough time has elapsed. You can use the fast-forward feature to advance the time by 2-minute intervals if the video is not yet available. Then click again on **Patient Care** and **Nurse-Client Interactions** to refresh the screen.)

2. What two factors did you discover that might contribute to Kathryn Doyle's risk for a fall?

3. Kathryn Doyle has a history of osteoporosis. This condition results in a loss of bone

   _____.

→ • Click on **Kardex** and review the activity orders for Kathryn Doyle.

4. What does the Kardex say about Kathryn Doyle's activity orders?

5. Kathryn Doyle has indicated a lack of interest in ambulation. What relationship exists between activity level and the development of osteoporosis?

6. When you assist Kathryn Doyle to get up from the bed to sit in the chair, you should perform several actions in a particular sequence. Listed below are the actions you would need to take after positioning the chair next to the bed. Number these steps to show the order in which you would perform them.

Action	**Order of Action**
_____ Assist her to sit.	a. 1
_____ Put firm-soled slippers on her feet.	b. 2
_____ Place a transfer belt around her waist.	c. 3
_____ Ask her whether she is dizzy.	d. 4
_____ Sit her up on the side of the bed.	e. 5
_____ Allow a couple of minutes for her to dangle.	f. 6
_____ Allow a couple of minutes for her blood pressure to stabilize.	g. 7
	h. 8
_____ Help her to a standing position.	i. 9
_____ Tell her what you are going to do.	
	j. 10
_____ Lower the bed.	
	k. 11
_____ Assist her to the chair, gripping the transfer belt.	

 • Click on **Return to Room 503** and then on **MAR**. Review Kathryn Doyle's MAR.

7. What medication is Kathryn Doyle receiving that could contribute to a fall? Why? (*Hint:* To check her medications for side effects, consult the Drug Guide [click on **Drug**] or use your pharmacology book or nursing drug handbook.)

Read about anemia in your medical-surgical textbook.

8. How can an anemic condition be a factor in a fall for an elderly person?

Nursing Care of the Elderly: Psychosocial Care

 Reading Assignment: Promoting Healthy Adaptation to Aging (Chapter 13)
Common Psychosocial Care Problems of the Elderly
(Chapter 41)

Patients: Clarence Hughes, Medical-Surgical Floor, Room 404
William Jefferson, Skilled Nursing Floor, Room 501
Kathryn Doyle, Skilled Nursing Floor, Room 503

Objectives:

1. Identify the various types of elder abuse.
2. Determine factors that indicate an elderly person needs assistance.
3. Assess developmental level factors in the elderly.
4. Describe factors that might indicate depression in the elderly.

Exercise 1

 CD-ROM Activity—Abuse, Depression, and Need for Assistance

🕐 30 minutes

- Sign in to work at Pacific View Regional Hospital on the Skilled Nursing Floor for Period of Care 3. (*Note:* If you are already in the virtual hospital from a previous exercise, click on **Leave the Floor** and then **Restart the Program** to get to the sign-in window.)
- From the Patient List, select Kathryn Doyle (Room 503).
- Click on **Go to Nurses' Station**.
- Click on **Chart** and then on **503**.
- Click on the **Nurse's Notes** and review the note regarding the incident with a family member.
- Click on **Consultations** and **Nursing Admission** and review the data.

1. Depression is often overlooked in the elderly. The physician has ordered a psychiatric nurse consult for Kathryn Doyle. What information have you found in her chart that might contribute to depression for Kathryn Doyle?

→ • Click on **Return to Nurses' Station** and then on **503** to visit Kathryn Doyle.
   • Click on **Patient Care** and then on **Nurse-Client Interactions**.
   • Select and view the video titled **1505: Assessment—Elder Abuse**. (*Note:* Check the virtual clock to see whether enough time has elapsed. You can use the fast-forward feature to advance the time by 2-minute intervals if the video is not yet available. Then click again on **Patient Care** and **Nurse-Client Interactions** to refresh the screen.)

2. Which of the following assessment findings for depression does Kathryn Doyle exhibit? Select all that apply. (*Hint:* Base your answers on the video interaction you just observed, as well as your review of the chart.)

_____ Fatigue

_____ Envy/criticism of others

_____ Appetite changes

_____ "Not feeling good"

_____ Sleep pattern changes

_____ Poor outlook on life

_____ Headaches

_____ Memory impairment

_____ Feelings of worthlessness/helplessness

3. The psychiatric nurse specialist suggests that Kathryn Doyle be started on an

_____ of the _____ type.

4. The primary responsibility of the nurse when a patient is started on this type of medication

is to _____.

5. Kathryn Doyle has not been taken to the dentist to have her dentures fixed for a very long

   time, and she is having trouble eating. This could be considered as _____
   on the part of her son.

6. Kathryn Doyle's son will not let her cook, clean, or manage her own money. She has indicated that she feels useless. These actions on the part of her son might be considered what
   type of abuse?

7. After a spouse dies, what signs would indicate that the surviving elderly spouse needs help
   and perhaps should not live alone? Select all that apply.

   _____ Frequently unable to find the right words

   _____ Forgetfulness

   _____ Withdrawn from others

   _____ Suspicious of others

   _____ Confused about medications

   _____ Watching a lot of TV

   _____ Frequent falls

   _____ Social isolation

   _____ Not paying bills

Exercise 2

CD-ROM Activity—Therapeutic Communication and Medication

30 minutes

- Sign in to work at Pacific View Regional Hospital on the Skilled Nursing Floor for Period of
  Care 3. (*Note:* If you are already in the virtual hospital from a previous exercise, click on
  Leave the Floor and then **Restart the Program** to get to the sign-in window.)
- From the Patient List, select William Jefferson (Room 501).
- Click on **Go to Nurses' Station**.
- Click on **MAR** and select tab **501**. Review William Jefferson's prescribed drugs.

  1. The physician has prescribed _____ for William Jefferson's
     Alzheimer's disease.

- Click on **Return to Nurses' Station** and then click on the **Drug** icon in the lower left corner
  of the screen. Scroll to the drug you identified in question 1 and read about it.

2. Below is a list of the possible side effects of the drug that has been prescribed for William Jefferson's Alzheimer's disease. Match each side effect with its degree of frequency.

Side Effect	Frequency of Side Effect
_____ Syncope	a. Frequent
_____ Nausea	b. Occasional
_____ Insomnia	c. Rare
_____ Tremor	
_____ Diarrhea	
_____ Anorexia	
_____ Hypertension	
_____ Anxiety	
_____ Headache	
_____ Confusion	

3. Does William Jefferson have other problems that this drug could exacerbate? If so, explain.

4. What would you teach William Jefferson and his wife about this drug?

→ • Click on **Return to Nurses' Station**.
   • Click on **501** to visit William Jefferson.
   • Click on **Patient Care** and perform a neurologic and mental status assessment by clicking first on **Head & Neck** and then on each of the subcategories in the green boxes.
   • After you have finished the assessment, click on **Nurse-Client Interactions**.
   • Select and view the video titled **1525: Living with Alzheimer's**. (*Note:* Check the virtual clock to see whether enough time has elapsed. You can use the fast-forward feature to advance the time by 2-minute intervals if the video is not yet available. Then click again on **Patient Care** and **Nurse-Client Interactions** to refresh the screen.)

5. What is the first question the student nurse asks after sitting down?

6. The question you identified above is an example of what therapeutic communication technique?

7. William Jefferson says that when he can't remember, it makes him feel stupid. What does the student nurse say in response to this? What therapeutic technique is she using here?

8. What is the primary goal of psychosocial interventions for the confused or disoriented elder?

9. What are the other principles of care for the cognitively impaired elder?

Exercise 3

  CD-ROM Activity—Developmental Tasks and Health Promotion

30 minutes

- Sign in to work at Pacific View Regional Hospital on the Medical-Surgical Floor for Period of Care 1. (*Note:* If you are already in the virtual hospital from a previous exercise, click on **Leave the Floor** and then **Restart the Program** to get to the sign-in window.)
- From the Patient List, select Clarence Hughes (Room 404).
- Click on **Go to Nurses' Station**.
- Click on **Chart** and then on **404**.
- Click on the tab for **Nursing Admission** and review the data.

1. Clarence Hughes is _____ years old. He is in Erikson's stage of

    _____ and appears to be in _____.

2. What information tells you that Clarence Hughes is in the positive side of this developmental phase?

3. In contrast to Clarence Hughes, Kathryn Doyle is in the _____ phase of this developmental level. (*Hint:* Base your answer on what you learned about Kathryn Doyle in Exercise 1 of this lesson.)

4. What data from Exercise 1 support your answer to question 3?

5. Based on the data you have collected on Clarence Hughes, indicate how each of the following actions applies in his case.

Actions	How It Applies
_____ Obtains a flu shot each year	a. Health promoting for him
_____ Wears a seat belt when in the car	b. Risk to his health
_____ Obtains a prostate exam	c. Not done by him
_____ Smokes cigarettes	
_____ Drinks alcohol occasionally	
_____ Watches TV most of the time	
_____ Performs self-testicular exam	
_____ Keeps weight within a normal range	
_____ Takes a vitamin-mineral supplement daily	
_____ Uses medications for glaucoma regularly	

6. After his rehabilitation period, what health promotion behaviors would you recommend to Clarence Hughes?

7. What health promotion behaviors would you recommend for Kathryn Doyle?

LESSON 8

Loss, Grief, and the Dying Patient

 Reading Assignment: Cultural and Spiritual Aspects of Patient Care (Chapter 14)
Loss, Grief, the Dying Patient, and Palliative Care (Chapter 15)

Patient: Goro Oishi, Skilled Nursing Floor, Room 505

Objectives:

1. Describe the stages of grief and of dying, with their associated behaviors and feelings.
2. Discuss the concepts of hospice care.
3. List common signs of impending death.
4. Recognize the responsibilities of the nurse related to postmortem care.

Exercise 1

 CD-ROM Activity—Advance Directives

30 minutes

- Sign in to work at Pacific View Regional Hospital on the Skilled Nursing Floor for Period of Care 1. (*Note:* If you are already in the virtual hospital from a previous exercise, click on **Leave the Floor** and then **Restart the Program** to get to the sign-in window.)
- From the Patient List, select Goro Oishi (Room 505).
- Click on **Get Report** and read the report.
- Click on **Go to Nurses' Station**.
- Click on **Chart** and then on **505**.
- Click on and read the **History and Physical**, **Admissions**, and **Physician's Orders**.

1. Why was Goro Oishi admitted to the hospital, and what is his current status?

2. What plans for care are identified in the History and Physical?

3. Does Goro Oishi have an advance directive?

4. Goro Oishi's plan of care is a form of assisted suicide.
   a. True
   b. False

5. Which of the following are usually present in hospice care? Select all that apply.

   _____ Focus on symptom management

   _____ Focus on comfort care

   _____ Care for the family

   _____ Rigorous treatment of infection

   _____ Rigorous invasive measures to prolong life

   _____ Care in the hospital, home, or other facility

6. The type of care delivered within a hospice program is often termed

   _____.

7. Considering Goro Oishi's condition, his advance directive, and the principles of hospice/palliative care, which of the following nursing actions would be appropriate for him during this shift? Select all that apply.

   _____ Instill lubricating eye drops

   _____ Prepare to insert feeding tube

   _____ Assess IV site every 2 hours

   _____ Monitor oxygen saturation

   _____ Monitor urine output via Foley catheter

   _____ Medicate for nausea

   _____ Turn and reposition every 2 hours

   _____ Assess skin for pressure areas every 2 hours

   _____ Medicate for elevated temperature

_____ Get him up to the chair once a shift

_____ Talk to him as care is provided

_____ Give him a bed bath

_____ Seek an order for treating constipation

_____ Provide urinary catheter care

 • Click on **Return to Nurses' Station** and then on **505** to go to the patient's room.
• Inside the room, click on **Patient Care** and then on **Nurse-Client Interactions**.
• Select and view the video titled **0735: Assessment—Family**. (*Note:* Check the virtual clock to see whether enough time has elapsed. You can use the fast-forward feature to advance the time by 2-minute intervals if the video is not yet available. Then click again on **Patient Care** and **Nurse-Client Interactions** to refresh the screen.)

8. What do you think Mrs. Oishi means when she tells the nurse that she wishes her son would accept his father's wishes?

 • Again, click on **Patient Care** and then on **Nurse-Client Interactions**.
• To complete the remaining questions in this exercise, you need to view two more nurse-client video interactions: **0745: Intervention—Clarification** and **0750: Family Conflict—Plan of Care**. (*Note:* Check the virtual clock to see whether enough time has elapsed. You can use the fast-forward feature to advance the time by 2-minute intervals if the video is not yet available. Then click again on **Patient Care** and **Nurse-Client Interactions** to refresh the screen.)

9. Match each Oishi family member with his or her present stage of grief.

Family Member	**Stage of Grief**
_____ Mrs. Oishi (patient's wife)	a. Shock and disbelief
_____ Kiyoshi (patient's youngest son)	b. Protest
_____ Namishi (patient's oldest son)	c. Disorganization
	d. Reorganization

10. An advance directive:
   a. states the patient's wishes in case of illness.
   b. spells out the patient's wishes for health care when patient is unable to indicate his or her choice.
   c. legally appoints a person to carry out one's wishes.
   d. is aimed at prolonging life.

11. What are three advantages of having an advance directive in place?

Exercise 2

 CD-ROM Activity—Signs of Deterioration

 30 minutes

In addition to an advance directive, a patient may have a signed durable power of attorney. Mrs. Oishi has the durable power of attorney for health care for Goro Oishi.

- Sign in to work at Pacific View Regional Hospital on the Skilled Nursing Floor for Period of Care 2. (*Note:* If you are already in the virtual hospital from a previous exercise, click on **Leave the Floor** and then **Restart the Program** to get to the sign-in window.)
- From the Patient List, select Goro Oishi (Room 505).
- Click on **Get Report** and read the report.
- Click on **Go to Nurses' Station**.
- Click on **505** and then on **Take Vital Signs**.

1. Record Goro Oishi's current vital signs below.

    BP ___173/89___ SpO2 ___86___ T ___100.8___ HR ___84___ RR ___20___

 • Click on and read the **Initial Observations** and the **Clinical Alerts**.
- Click on **EPR** and then on **Login**. Select **505** as the Patient and **Vital Signs** as the Category.
- Enter Goro Oishi's vital signs in the appropriate time column.
- Using the arrow at the bottom of the screen, scroll back to compare vital signs from previous times.

2. Complete the table below by entering Goro Oishi's vital signs from the EPR for the days and times specified.

Assessment of Vital Sign Trends

	Mon 1545	Tues 0800	Wed 1130
BP	136/80	142/72	173/83
SpO$_2$	95	93	86
T	98	98.8	100.8
HR	68	78	84
RR	20	18	20

3. What changes or trends do you see in the vital signs?

BP ↑

SpO$_2$ ↓

T ↑

HR ↑

RR Same

4. Which of the following are physical signs of approaching death? Select all that apply.

___✓___ Temperature rises

___✓___ Heart rate rises

_____ Heart rate drops

_____ Blood pressure rises

___✓___ Blood pressure drops

___✓___ Respirations become irregular

___✓___ Extremities become mottled, cool, and dusky

5. Considering the fact that Goro Oishi is comatose and unresponsive, it is impossible for the family to interact with him. What should the nurse caution the family to be careful about when in Goro Oishi's room?

That he may be unresponsive but hearing is the last to go.

- Click on **Exit EPR** to return to the patient's room.
- Click on **Patient Care** and then on **Nurse-Client Interactions**.
- Select and view the video titled **1125: The Family Facing Death** and **1126: Supporting the Dying Patient**. (*Note:* Check the virtual clock to see whether enough time has elapsed. You can use the fast-forward feature to advance the time by 2-minute intervals if the video is not yet available. Then click again on **Patient Care** and **Nurse-Client Interactions** to refresh the screen.)

6. Does the younger son seem open to hearing any discussion of Goro Oishi's beliefs?

   NO, he thinks it's a loss cause and wont do any good and its his mothers fault.

7. When working with the Oishi family, what communication techniques can be used to assist them in dealing with the situation?

   active listening, provide support and empathy.

8. The nurse's interaction with Goro Oishi's son provides him with information that enables him to accept his father's death.
   a. True
   b. False *(circled)*

- Click on **Patient Care** and then **Nurse-Client Interactions**.
- Select and view the video titled **1128: The Medical Power of Attorney**. (*Note:* Check the virtual clock to see whether enough time has elapsed. You can use the fast-forward feature to advance the time by 2-minute intervals if the video is not yet available. Then click again on **Patient Care** and **Nurse-Client Interactions** to refresh the screen.)

9. Which of the following does Mrs. Oishi try to explain to her son? Select all that apply.

   ✓ She was chosen by her husband as his "agent" in case he reached the end of his life.

   _____ She loves her husband and wants him to live.

   _____ She wishes to respect his (Goro Oishi's) wishes.

   ✓ She wishes to allow her husband to die with dignity.

   _____ There is no way that her husband's condition will allow him to live.

10. Goro Oishi's son's objection to the advance directive does not invalidate it.
    a. True *(circled)*
    b. False

Exercise 3

CD-ROM Activity—Signs of Impending Death

15 minutes

- Sign in to work at Pacific View Regional Hospital on the Skilled Nursing Floor for Period of Care 3. (*Note:* If you are already in the virtual hospital from a previous exercise, click on **Leave the Floor** and then **Restart the Program** to get to the sign-in window.)
- From the Patient List, select Goro Oishi (Room 505).
- Click on **Get Report** and read the report.
- Click on **Go to Nurses' Station** and then on **505** to go to the patient's room.
- Read the **Initial Observations**.

1. A change noted in the Initial Observations that indicates Goro Oishi's kidneys have shut down is <u>NO urine output.</u> for the last 4 hours.

→ • Click on **Take Vital Signs**.

2. What are Goro Oishi's current vital signs?

BP <u>80/58</u>   SpO$_2$ <u>80</u>   T <u>99.5</u>   HR <u>96</u>   RR <u>10</u>

3. Compare these current vital signs with the last ones you measured. What changes do you see in the vital signs now?
   ↓ BP
   ↓ oxygen
   ↓ temp
   ↑ HR
   ↓ RR

→ • Click on **Patient Care** and then on **Nurse-Client Interactions**.
- Select and view the video titled **1500: Patient Decline**.
- Next, select and view the video titled **1505: Meeting the Spiritual Needs**. (*Note:* Check the virtual clock to see whether enough time has elapsed. You can use the fast-forward feature to advance the time by 2-minute intervals if the video is not yet available. Then click again on **Patient Care** and **Nurse-Client Interactions** to refresh the screen.)

4. What change is happening to Goro Oishi?
   he is having a hard time breathing and health is decreasing.

5. The family requests that <u>buddist munk</u> be called.

6. Goro Oishi's vital signs have ceased, and the nurse has called the physician. Which of the following should she also do now? Select all that apply. (*Hint:* See pages 204-206 of your textbook.)

_____✓ Ask the family members whether they wish to help prepare the body.

_____✓ Allow the family time alone with the patient.

_____✓ Remove tubes and cleanse the body.

_____ Prepare the body for the mortuary or coroner.

_____ Ask family members whether they want the nurse to stay with them while they view the body.

_____✓ Offer condolences.

LESSON 9

Pain, Comfort, and Sleep

 Reading Assignment: Cultural and Spiritual Aspects of Patient Care (Chapter 14)
Pain, Comfort, and Sleep (Chapter 31)
Complementary and Alternative Therapies (Chapter 32)

Patients: Clarence Hughes, Medical-Surgical Floor, Room 404
Pablo Rodriguez, Medical-Surgical Floor, Room 405
Kathryn Doyle, Skilled Nursing Floor, Room 503

Objectives:

1. Recall the parameters for assessment of pain.
2. Discuss the physiologic responses to pain.
3. Identify comfort measures to help relieve pain and promote rest.
4. Determine precautions for giving various analgesics.
5. Develop awareness of cultural and individual responses to pain.
6. Choose interventions to help the patient sleep and rest in the hospital.

Exercise 1

 CD-ROM Activity—Pain Assessment

⏱ 30 minutes

- Sign in to work at Pacific View Regional Hospital on the Medical-Surgical Floor for Period of Care 1. (*Note:* If you are already in the virtual hospital from a previous exercise, click on **Leave the Floor** and then **Restart the Program** to get to the sign-in window.)
- From the Patient List, select Clarence Hughes (Room 404).
- Click on **Get Report** and read the report.
- Click on **Go to Nurses' Station** and then on **404**.
- Read the **Initial Observations** and click on **Clinical Alerts**.
- Click on **Take Vital Signs** and record them below.

1. What are Clarence Hughes' current vital signs?

   BP _____ SpO$_2$ _____ T _____ HR _____ RR _____ Pain _____

→ • Click on **EPR** and **Login**. Choose **404** as the Patient and Vital Signs as the Category. Document the vital signs.

2. Are there any appreciable differences between Clarence Hughes' current vital signs and the previous vital signs?

3. Why is it important to measure the vital signs as part of the pain assessment?

4. When assessing pain, what four factors should be assessed?

5. Review Clarence Hughes' condition and complaints of pain. Which of the following pain types is he most likely experiencing?
   a. Chronic pain
   b. Nociceptive pain
   c. Neuropathic pain
   d. Phantom pain

→ • Click on **Exit EPR** and then on **MAR**. Select tab **404** for Clarence Hughes' MAR.
   • Scroll through the MAR, noting the medication orders.

6. The medication ordered for Clarence Hughes' pain is _____.

→ • Click on **Return to Room 404.**
   • Click on **Chart** and then **404**.
   • Select the chart tab for **Expired MARs**.

7. According to the expired MARs, how frequently has Clarence Hughes been receiving the pain pills?

8. Clarence Hughes is at risk for what problem(s) while taking this medication?

→ • Click on **Return to Room 404**
   • Click on **EPR** and then **Login**. Choose **404** as the Patient and **Gastrointestinal** as the Category.

9. Clarence Hughes had his last bowel movement _____.

10. The notes you have read indicate that his knee and lower leg are swollen. How does this affect the pain level?

11. When Clarence Hughes' leg is not in the CPM machine, which of the following adjunctive measures might be used to decrease his pain? Select all that apply.

   _____ Application of heat

   _____ Application of cold

   _____ Elevation of the leg and knee

   _____ Distraction with a book, TV, or visitor

   _____ Loud, lively music

   _____ Favorite music softly played

   _____ Imagery exercise

   _____ Relaxation exercise

   _____ Chiropractic manipulation

It is always important to perform an assessment of spirituality, coping ability, and cultural preferences when a patient is admitted. What the assessment reveals should be woven into the plan of care.

→ • Click on **Exit EPR**. Now click on **Chart** and then on **404**.
   • Select the **Nursing Admission** and review this record.

12. Does Clarence Hughes have any particular spiritual beliefs or practices? If so, what are they?

13. Does Clarence Hughes indicate that he has good coping skills?

14. Does he have any special cultural practices?

Clarence Hughes doesn't have trouble sleeping at home, but in the hospital he finds uninterrupted sleep difficult. The physician has ordered medication to help him sleep.

→ • Click on **Return to Room 404** and then on **MAR**. Find the medication that is prescribed for sleep.

15. The physician has ordered _____ to help Clarence Hughes sleep. This

drug should be given _____ before he wishes to fall sleep. This drug is

classified as a _____.

Exercise 2

CD-ROM Activity—Chronic Pain

15 minutes

• Sign in to work at Pacific View Regional Hospital on the Medical-Surgical Floor for Period of Care 1. (*Note:* If you are already in the virtual hospital from a previous exercise, click on **Leave the Floor** and then **Restart the Program** to get to the sign-in window.)
• From the Patient List, select Pablo Rodriguez (Room 405).
• Click on **Get Report** and read the report.
• Click on **Go to Nurses' Station**.
• Click on **405** and then on **Take Vital Signs**.

1. Pablo Rodriguez has metastatic carcinoma of the lung and has been admitted with nausea, vomiting, dehydration, and poor pain control. What are his vital signs at this time?

BP _____ SpO$_2$ _____ T _____ HR _____ RR _____ Pain _____

2. What type of pain do you think Pablo Rodriguez is experiencing?

→ • Click on **MAR** and note the the medications Pablo Rodriguez is receiving.

3. What is ordered for pain management for Pablo Rodriguez?

4. Pablo Rodriguez is receiving _____ IV as an adjunctive medication to help control his pain.

➤ • Click on **Return to Room 405** and then on the **Drug** icon in the lower left corner of the screen.
   • Scroll to the medication you listed in question 4.

5. How do you think this medication helps decrease pain?

➤ • Click on **Return to Room 405** and then click on **Chart**.
   • Select the **Nursing Admission** and scroll to the sections on spiritual, cultural, and coping assessment.

6. What does Pablo Rodriguez say about his coping ability?

7. Where does he say his pain is located? How does he describe his pain?

8. Pablo Rodriguez's spiritual orientation is _____, and he feels that

_____.

9. If Pablo Rodriguez were able to take PO medications, what other type of adjunctive medications might help with his pain control?

10. Listed below are interventions used to help relieve pain. Match each specific intervention with its type.

Intervention	Type of Measure or Therapy
_____ Reposition every hour	a. Adjunctive measure
_____ Keep lights low	b. Comfort measure
_____ Acupuncture	c. Complementary or alternative therapy
_____ Tricyclic antidepressants	
_____ Relaxation exercises	
_____ Imagery exercises	
_____ Change bed linens	
_____ Biofeedback	
_____ Soft music	
_____ Aromatherapy	

→ • Scroll to the Rest and Activity portion of the Nursing Admission.

11. To help Pablo Rodriguez sleep, you would make sure that there are

_____ available to help him get comfortable.

12. Is there a sleeping medication ordered for Pablo Rodriguez?

Exercise 3

 CD-ROM Activity—Factors that Influence Perception of Pain

 20 minutes

• Sign in to work at Pacific View Regional Hospital on the Skilled Nursing Floor for Period of Care 2. (*Note:* If you are already in the virtual hospital from a previous exercise, click on **Leave the Floor** and then **Restart the Program** to get to the sign-in window.)
• From the Patient List, select Kathryn Doyle (Room 503).
• Click on **Get Report** and read the report.
• Click on **Go to Nurses' Station**.
• Click on **EPR** and then on **Login**.
• Select **503** as the Patient and **Vital Signs** as the Category, Scroll backward in time through the vital signs findings.

1. Kathryn Doyle's pain has ranged from _____ to _____ on a scale of 1-10.

→ • Click on **Exit EPR** and then on **503**.
   • Click on **Patient Care** and then on **Nurse-Client Interactions**.
   • Select and view the video titled **1130: The Unexpected Event**. (*Note:* Check the virtual clock to see whether enough time has elapsed. You can use the fast-forward feature to advance the time by 2-minute intervals if the video is not yet available. Then click again on **Patient Care** and **Nurse-Client Interactions** to refresh the screen.)

2. What does Kathryn Doyle seem to be experiencing related to this interaction and the events that have occurred?

3. Which of the following factors do you think might make the perception of pain worse? Select all that apply.

_____ Pleasant visitors

_____ Fear

_____ Excessive noise

_____ Clean, quiet environment

_____ Anxiety

_____ Stress

_____ Inadequate sleep

_____ Attentive nurse

_____ Constipation

→ • Click on **MAR** and note the medications ordered for Kathryn Doyle.

4. What medication is ordered for pain for Kathryn Doyle?

5. Is there an adjunctive medication ordered that will help relieve her pain?

6. Oxycodone tends to be constipating. What dietary recommendations would you make to help prevent Kathryn Doyle from experiencing constipation?

7. Kathryn Doyle has _____ ordered to help prevent constipation. (*Hint:* See the MAR.)

8. How does this medication work to help prevent constipation?

➤ • Click on **EPR** and then on **Login**. Select **503** as the Patient and **Gastrointestinal** as the Category.

9. Kathryn Doyle had her last bowel movement _____ and

_____ (is/is not) experiencing constipation.

10. Does Kathryn Doyle have anything ordered to help her sleep? If so, what?

➤ • Click on **Exit EPR** and then on **Chart**.
   • Select the chart for **503** and click on **Nursing Admission** tab. Scroll down to the section on Rest and Activity.

11. What does Kathryn Doyle do in preparation for sleep?

12. How might this activity interfere with her ability to sleep?

LESSON 10 —————————————————

Activity, Mobility, and Skin Care

——————————————————————————————

Reading Assignment: Infection Prevention and Control in the Hospital and Home
(Chapter 17)
Lifting, Moving, and Positioning Patients (Chapter 18)
Assisting with Hygiene, Personal Care, Skin Care, and the
Prevention of Pressure Ulcers (Chapter 19)
Promoting Musculoskeletal Function (Chapter 39)

Patients: Harry George, Medical-Surgical Floor, Room 401
Clarence Hughes, Medical-Surgical Floor, Room 404
Patricia Newman, Medical-Surgical Floor, Room 406

Objectives:

1. Recognize areas of pressure that occur with different patient positions.
2. Recall risk factors that contribute to the formation of pressure ulcers.
3. Discuss the effects of immobility on the body's systems.
4. Assist patients to use devices that promote mobility.

Exercise 1

 CD-ROM Activity—Complications of Immobility

 30 minutes

- Sign in to work at Pacific View Regional Hospital on the Medical-Surgical Floor for Period of Care 2. (*Note:* If you are already in the virtual hospital from a previous exercise, click on **Leave the Floor** and then **Restart the Program** to get to the sign-in window.)
- From the Patient List, select Clarence Hughes (Room 404).
- Click on **Get Report** and note pertinent information given in the report.
- Click on **Go to Nurses' Station** and then on **404**.
- Read the **Initial Observations** and the **Clinical Alerts**.
- Click on **Chart** and then on **404**. Select the **Physician's Orders**.

1. Clarence Hughes had a left total knee arthroplasty (replacement) on Monday. What are the current activity orders for Clarence Hughes?

2. Clarence Hughes will be in a supine or semi-Fowler's position during the day in order to use the CPM device; thus he will not be able to turn to his side. However, at night he may turn to the right side. Below, match the pressure areas related to a supine position and those related to a side-lying position.

Pressure Area	Position
_____ Sacrum/coccyx	a. Supine position
_____ Occiput	b. Side-lying position
_____ Dorsal/thoracic area	
_____ Ischial tuberosity	
_____ Posterior knee	
_____ Malleolus	
_____ Lateral knee	
_____ Ilium	
_____ Trochanter	
_____ Shoulder	
_____ Elbow	
_____ Heel	
_____ Shoulder blade	

3. When an area of redness is observed after turning a patient, what is the appropriate action?

_____ Massage the area.

_____ Reassess the area in 30-45 minutes.

_____ Immediately check to see whether the area will blanch.

_____ Apply a hot pack to the area.

4. You turn Clarence Hughes from a side-lying to a supine position during the night, and you notice a reddened area on the right hip. The area does not blanch when you go back to check on it in an hour. You should chart that he has a stage _____ pressure ulcer.

5. If a stage 1 pressure ulcer has formed, which of the following should you do?
   a. Leave the area open to the air.
   b. Apply a hydrocolloid dressing.
   c. Apply a gauze dressing.
   d. Apply a transparent film dressing.

6. What are the purposes of using continuous passive motion after joint replacement?

7. Clarence Hughes' new knee and its limited range of motion put him at risk for a fall. When he gets up to ambulate, you would teach him to do which of the following? Select all that apply.

   _____ Sit for a minute or two before standing.

   _____ Stand still until any dizziness passes before beginning to walk.

   _____ Wear firm-soled slippers.

   _____ Lean slightly forward while using the walker.

   _____ Maintain good, upright posture while ambulating.

   _____ Ambulate only with someone holding on to him.

8. Because Clarence Hughes has had a knee joint replacement, he is at risk for neurovascular impairment. You should perform a neurovascular assessment on him every shift. Based on

   Clarence Hughes' age, the capillary refill in his toes should be _____.

9. Describe how you would check sensation when performing your neurovascular assessment.

10. What are the four effects of immobility on the musculoskeletal system? Select all that apply.

   _____ Renal stones

   _____ Venous stasis

   _____ Decreased muscle mass and muscle tension

   _____ Negative nitrogen balance

   _____ Ischemia and necrosis of tissue

   _____ Shortening of muscle

_____ Loss of calcium from bone matrix

_____ Decrease in bone weight

_____ Decreased independence

11. Because of the immobility caused by his surgical procedure, Clarence Hughes is at risk for

the cardiovascular-respiratory complication called _____.

12. Clarence Hughes will be transported to the radiology department for a ventilation-perfusion scan. He will be transported by wheelchair. A major safety precaution when transferring a patient into or out of a wheelchair is to:
   a. place the chair to the left of the patient, who is seated on the bed.
   b. place the chair to the right of the patient, who is seated on the bed.
   c. move the leg extensions on the chair to the lowest position.
   d. check to see that the wheel locks are engaged.

Read in your textbook about the complication you identified in question 11.

→ • Click on **Return to Room 404**.
   • Click on **Patient Care** and then on **Chest**.
   • One at a time, click on each subcategory (the green boxes) of the chest assessment.

13. Based on the change-of-shift report, the Initial Observations, the Clinical Alert, and your chest assessment, Clarence Hughes has shown which signs and symptoms of the complication you identified in question 11? Select all that apply.

_____ Leaning forward

_____ Diaphoresis

_____ Coughing

_____ Shortness of breath

_____ Chest pain

_____ Anxiety

_____ Tachypnea

_____ Production of frothy sputum

Exercise 2

 CD-ROM Activity—Pressure Ulcer Risk and Infection

⏱ 30 minutes

   • Sign in to work at Pacific View Regional Hospital on the Medical-Surgical Floor for Period of Care 1. (*Note:* If you are already in the virtual hospital from a previous exercise, click on **Leave the Floor** and then **Restart the Program** to get to the sign-in window.)
   • From the Patient List, select Harry George (Room 401).

- Click on **Get Report** and review the report.
- Click on **Go to Nurses' Station** and then on **401**.
- Read the **Initial Observations** and **Clinical Alerts** notes.
- Click on **Chart** and then on **401**. Select the **Physician's Orders**.

1. What are the activity and positioning orders for Harry George?

2. When elevating Harry George's foot on pillows, you must be very careful to protect the

   _____ from pressure.

→ • Click on **History and Physical** and read through the form.

3. From the information in the History and Physical, what would you expect Harry George's nutritional status to be?

4. Which of the following factors cause a patient to be at greater risk for a pressure ulcer? Select all that apply.

   _____ Continued diaphoresis

   _____ Obesity

   _____ Weight loss

   _____ Incontinence

   _____ Bed rest

   _____ Dehydration

   _____ Confusion

   _____ Edema

   _____ Poor nutrition

5. Considering the data you have obtained, how many risk factors does Harry George have for developing a pressure ulcer? What are they?

➡ • Click on **Physician's Notes** and determine what organism has caused the infection in Harry George's foot.

6. The organism causing the infection in Harry George's foot is

_____.

➡ • Click on **Return to Room 401** and then on **Patient Care**.
   • Perform a focused assessment on Harry George's **Lower Extremities**.

7. Below, record your findings from the focused assessment of Harry George's lower extremities.

Focused Assessment—Lower Extremities

Integumentary

Musculoskeletal

Vascular

Neurologic

➡ • Click on **EPR** and then on **Login**.
   • Select **401** as the Patient. Using the drop-down Category menu, select each appropriate category and document the assessment data you just obtained from Harry George.

8. The physician has ordered dressing changes for Harry George's foot. This procedure requires the use of standard precautions. Which of the following protective barrier items will be required to perform this dressing change? Select all that apply.

_____ Gloves

_____ Gown

_____ Mask

_____ Goggles

_____ Biohazard discard bag

_____ Private room

9. There are special criteria for transmission-based precautions in the hospital. Harry George's

wound would require _____ precautions.

10. When performing a dressing change for Harry George, you must adhere to principles of aseptic technique. Indicate the actions that adhere to aseptic principles while performing this dressing change. Select all that apply.

_____ Do not use dressings that have been opened but left in the room.

_____ Set up the sterile field above your waist height.

_____ Open sterile pack wrappers away from the body.

_____ Open the sterile glove pack on your sterile field.

_____ Place the discard bag at the back edge of the sterile field.

_____ Once gloved, keep your hands in sight.

Exercise 3

CD-ROM Activity—Physical Therapy to Increase Mobility and Endurance

15 minutes

- Sign in to work at Pacific View Regional Hospital on the Medical-Surgical Floor for Period of Care 4. (*Note:* If you are already in the virtual hospital from a previous exercise, click on **Leave the Floor** and then **Restart the Program** to get to the sign-in window.)
- Click on **Chart** and then on **406**. Click on the **Consultations** tab and scroll to the PT/OT Consult. Read through the consultation notes. (*Remember:* You are not able to visit patients or administer medications during Period of Care 4. You are able to review patient records only.)

1. The plan states that Patricia Newman is to begin her pulmonary rehabilitation plan by

walking _____ minutes _____ times a day.

2. Patricia Newman is to walk _____ (independently/with assistance) for her activity plan.

3. What is the goal of the physical therapy program?

4. What parameters would need to be monitored when Patricia Newman starts the walking plan?

5. For which of the following activities does Patricia Newman require moderate assistance?

    _____ Bathing

    _____ Dressing

    _____ Toileting

    _____ Grooming

    _____ Eating

6. What might help Patricia Newman perform this daily activity task with less assistance?

7. The recommendations of the dietitian should be interwoven with the physical therapy plan. Why?

8. How might the exercise plan help prevent further bouts of pneumonia? (*Hint:* Use critical thinking for this question.)

Vital Signs, Health Status Assessment, and Data Collection

📖 **Reading Assignment:** Measuring Vital Signs (Chapter 21)
Assessing Health Status (Chapter 22)

Patients: Pablo Rodriguez, Medical-Surgical Floor, Room 405
Patricia Newman, Medical-Surgical Floor, Room 406

Objectives:

1. Recognize abnormal vital signs.
2. Recognize factors that can affect vital signs.
3. Identify abnormal findings from the physical assessment.
4. Identify priority areas of assessment for specific patients.
5. Determine components needed to perform a focused assessment for identified actual or potential problems.

Exercise 1

 CD-ROM Activity—Normal Versus Abnormal Vital Signs

 45 minutes

Observing trends in vital signs often gives clues to patient problems.

- Sign in to work at Pacific View Regional Hospital on the Medical-Surgical Floor for Period of Care 3. (*Note:* If you are already in the virtual hospital from a previous exercise, click on **Leave the Floor** and then **Restart the Program** to get to the sign-in window.)
- From the Patient List, select Pablo Rodriguez (Room 405).
- Click on **Get Report** and read the report.
- Click on **Go to Nurses' Station**.
- Click on **Chart** and then on **405**. Click on and review the **History and Physical**.
- Click on **Return to Nurses' Station** and then on **405** at the bottom of the screen.
- Click on **Take Vital Signs**. Record your findings in the top row of the table in question 2.
- Click on **EPR** and then **Login**. Choose **405** as the Patient and **Vital Signs** as the Category.
- Use the blue arrows at the bottom of the screen to scroll to the previous vital sign recordings.

1. Why has Pablo Rodriguez been admitted to the hospital?

2. In the table below, enter Pablo Rodriguez's current vital signs and his earlier vital signs from the EPR. Based on these findings, begin to analyze the trend of each vital sign.

Day	Time	BP	SpO$_2$	T	HR	RR	Pain
Current findings							
Wed							
Wed							
Wed							

3. From your analysis of the vital sign trends, what do you think is causing the changes in Pablo Rodriguez's heart rate and respiration?

4. The normal adult range for temperature is _____. The

normal pulse range for an adult is _____. The normal range for respira-

tions in the healthy adult is _____. The normal blood pressure for the

adult is _____.

5. Imagine you are applying the cuff of a manual sphygmomanometer to a patient's arm. From the list below, choose the appropriate steps for this procedure and number them in the correct order (from 1 to 4). If a step is incorrect (does not apply to the sequence), choose "e."

Step		**Order of Steps**
_____	Place the cuff ½ inch above the antecubital space.	a. 1
_____	Center the bladder over the brachial artery.	b. 2
_____	Verify that the cuff is 1½ times the diameter of the patient's arm.	c. 3
		d. 4
_____	Wrap the cuff smoothly but securely around the arm.	
_____	Place the cuff 1 to 2 inches above the antecubital space.	e. Not a correct step in the sequence!
_____	Obtain a cuff that is 21% larger than the patient's arm.	

6. You need to measure a patient's respirations. Why would it be a good idea to tell the patient you are measuring the pulse instead?

7. In the list below, select all choices that correctly finish the following statement. Taking an oral temperature would be contraindicated in a patient who:

_____ has been running a high temperature elevation.

_____ has had previous seizures.

_____ has just finished breakfast.

_____ is 7 years old.

_____ suffers from dementia.

_____ finished a cold soft drink 15 minutes ago.

_____ is newly postoperative.

_____ is a teenager with a leg fracture.

_____ is 2½ years old.

8. A rectal temperature is:
   a. 1 degree higher than an oral temperature.
   b. 1 degree lower than an oral temperature.

Exercise 2

 CD-ROM Activity—Assessment and Data Collection

 30 minutes

- Sign in to work at Pacific View Regional Hospital on the Medical-Surgical Floor for Period of Care 3. (*Note:* If you are already in the virtual hospital from a previous exercise, click on **Leave the Floor** and then **Restart the Program** to get to the sign-in window.)
- From the Patient List, select Pablo Rodriguez (Room 405).
- Click on **Go to Nurses' Station**.
- Click on **Chart** and then on **405**. Review the **History and Physical**.
- Click on **Return to Nurses' Station** and then on **405** at the bottom of the screen.
- Inside the room, click on **Patient Care** and then on **Physical Assessment**.
- Click on **Chest** and then on each subcategory (green boxes). Note your findings.
- Click on **Abdomen** and then on each subcategory (green boxes). Note your findings.

1. Below, record your findings from the focused assessment of Pablo Rodriguez.

Chest
  Integumentary

  Cardiovascular

  Respiratory

  Musculoskeletal

Abdomen
  Integumentary

  Musculoskeletal

  Gastrointestinal

 - Click on **Chart** and then on **405**.
- Select **Nurse's Notes** and read through the notes.

2. List indications of problems that should be considered when writing Pablo Rodriguez's care plan.

3. Which of the following would be appropriate nursing diagnoses, considering the data you have gathered from your physical assessment and the chart? Select all that apply.

_____ Ineffective airway clearance

_____ Constipation

_____ Impaired gas exchange

_____ Acute and chronic pain

_____ Noncompliance

_____ Nausea

_____ Anxiety

_____ Fear

_____ Impaired oral mucous membranes

4. Write one expected outcome for each of the nursing diagnoses you chose in question 3.

Exercise 3

 CD-ROM Activity—Data Collection

 30 minutes

- Sign in to work at Pacific View Regional Hospital on the Medical-Surgical Floor for Period of Care 3. (*Note:* If you are already in the virtual hospital from a previous exercise, click on **Leave the Floor** and then **Restart the Program** to get to the sign-in window.)
- From the Patient List, select Patricia Newman (Room 406).
- Click on **Get Report** and read the report.
- Click on **Go to Nurses' Station**.
- Click on **Chart** and then on **406**.
- Click on **Nursing Admission** and read the admission pages.

1. Why has Patricia Newman been admitted to the hospital?

2. What medications was Patricia Newman taking at home?

3. Patricia Newman says her religion is _____.

4. She states that she smokes _____ packs per day.

5. Does it appear that Patricia Newman practices "preventive health care" by obtaining immunizations, doing self-breast exams, and living a healthy lifestyle?

6. What does Patricia Newman indicate is her goal for this hospitalization?

7. Patricia Newman says her normal bowel pattern is _____.

8. What sleep aid does she say she uses?

9. Does she have any hearing or vision difficulties or impairments?

10. Describe Patricia Newman's family relationships.

Exercise 4

 CD-ROM Activity—Assessment

 15 minutes

- Sign in to work at Pacific View Regional Hospital on the Medical-Surgical Floor for Period of Care 3. (*Note:* If you are already in the virtual hospital from a previous exercise, click on **Leave the Floor** and then **Restart the Program** to get to the sign-in window.)
- From the Patient List, select Patricia Newman (Room 406).
- Click on **Go to Nurses' Station**.
- Click on **406** to go to the patient's room.
- Click on **Take Vital Signs**.

1. What are Patricia Newman's current vital sign measurements?

    BP _____ SpO$_2$ _____ T _____ HR _____ RR _____ Pain _____

2. When planning interventions to reduce Patricia Newman's temperature, which of the following may be included? Select all that apply.

    _____ Lower the environmental temperature.

    _____ Restrict fluid intake.

    _____ Provide a cold sponge bath.

    _____ Increase rate of air circulation.

    _____ Remove bed coverings.

3. How can Patricia Newman's blood pressure be best described?
    a. Normal
    b. Prehypertension
    c. Stage 1 hypertension
    d. Stage 2 hypertension

 - Click on **EPR** and **Login**.
- Select **406** as the Patient and **Vital Signs** as the Category.
- Review the vital sign patterns.

4. Patricia Newman's temperature recordings can best be described as:
    a. constant.
    b. intermittent.
    c. remittent.
    d. relapsing.

• Click on **Exit EPR**.

• Click **Patient Care** and then on **Nurse-Client Interactions**.

• Select and view the video titled **1500: Discharge Planning**. (*Note:* Check the virtual clock to see whether enough time has elapsed. You can use the fast-forward feature to advance the time by 2-minute intervals if the video is not yet available. Then click again on **Patient Care** and **Nurse-Client Interactions** to refresh the screen.)

5. What concerns and problems did you discover from the interaction?

Read in Chapter 22 of your textbook about assessment of the chest, heart, and lungs.

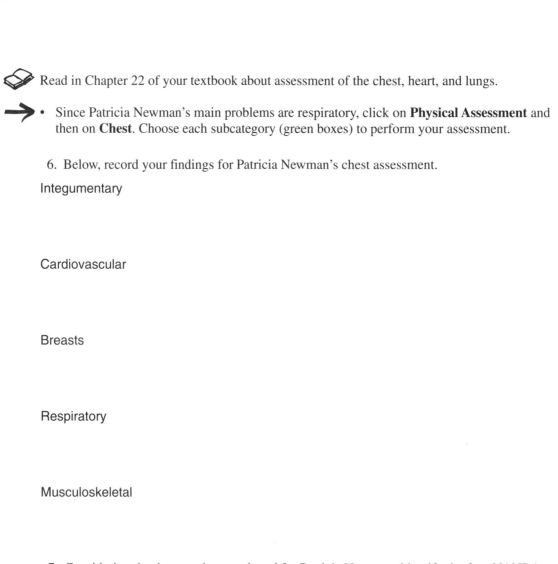 • Since Patricia Newman's main problems are respiratory, click on **Physical Assessment** and then on **Chest**. Choose each subcategory (green boxes) to perform your assessment.

6. Below, record your findings for Patricia Newman's chest assessment.

Integumentary

Cardiovascular

Breasts

Respiratory

Musculoskeletal

7. Considering the data you have gathered for Patricia Newman, identify the four NANDA nursing diagnoses that are priorities for her.

LESSON 12

Diagnostic Testing and Specimen Collection

 Reading Assignment: Diagnostic Tests and Specimen Collection (Chapter 24)

Patients: Harry George, Medical-Surgical Floor, Room 401
Piya Jordan, Medical-Surgical Floor, Room 403

Objectives:

1. Recognize abnormal laboratory values.
2. Provide pre- and posttest teaching.
3. Recall the proper patient preparation for various diagnostic tests.
4. Explain the purpose of various diagnostic tests.
5. Explain what to expect during various diagnostic tests.

Exercise 1

 CD-ROM Activity—Exploring Laboratory Values

30 minutes

- Sign in to work at Pacific View Regional Hospital on the Medical-Surgical Floor for Period of Care 3. (*Note:* If you are already in the virtual hospital from a previous exercise, click on Leave the Floor and then Restart the Program to get to the sign-in window.)
- From the Patient List, select Harry George (Room 401).
- Click on **Go to Nurses' Station** and then on **Chart**.
- Click on **401** for Harry George's chart; then select the **Physician's Orders**.

1. In the list below, identify the laboratory and diagnostic tests ordered for Harry George during this hospitalization. Select all that apply.

_____ Blood culture

_____ Ventilation perfusion scan

_____ CBC

_____ Chem 20

_____ Pulmonary function tests

_____ Bone scan

_____ Arterial blood gas

_____ Amylase and lipase

_____ Culture and sensitivity of wound

_____ KUB

_____ Clotting studies

_____ Folic acid level

_____ Alcohol level

_____ Chest x-ray

2. Discuss the relationship between Harry George's erythrocyte sedimentation rate and his admitting diagnosis.

3. When a blood chemistry panel is ordered, there is a requirement that _____

be withheld for _____ hours. (*Hint:* See page 407 in your textbook.)

→ • Click on the **Laboratory Reports** tab and scroll to the urinalysis results.

4. Below and on the next page, list the values for Harry George's urinalysis. Consider how these findings compare with the normals. Place an asterisk (*) after any finding that is not normal.

Color

Character

Specific gravity

Acetone, ketones

Glucose

Protein

Nitrite

Occult blood

pH

Micro cells
  Erythrocytes

  Leukocytes

  Bacteria

5. A wound culture was ordered for Harry George. Which of the following must the nurse do when obtaining a wound culture? (*Hint:* See Skill 24-5 on pages 428-430 in your textbook.)
   a. Cleanse the entire wound thoroughly.
   b. Insert the sterile swab into the area where drainage is occurring.
   c. Put on exam gloves before opening swab container.
   d. Swab at least two sites in the wound with one swab.

6. Harry George has a bone scan (radionuclide study) ordered for the left foot. Which of the following statements by the nurse are appropriate in the teaching process to prepare him for the scan? Select all that apply.

   _____ "You must be NPO for 8 hours prior to the scan."

   _____ "A radioactive substance will be injected into a vein."

   _____ "You will be isolated while the radioactive substance is in your body."

   _____ "There will be a delay before the scan while the radionuclide is absorbed by the bone."

   _____ "You will be asked to empty your bladder after the scan."

   _____ "You will be radioactive for 24 hours."

   _____ "You will not be radioactive or a danger to others in the vicinity."

• Still in the **Laboratory Reports** section of Harry George's chart, scroll back to find his Hematology results.

7. A complete blood count is often performed either to determine the presence of an infection in the body or to track whether treatment is clearing up an infection. When evaluating the CBC for signs of infection, you would check the number of

_____ and the number of _____.

Harry George's CBC values are _____ (normal; abnormal). (*Hint:* See Table 24-1 on page 406 in your textbook.)

➡ • Scroll to the Chemistry section of the Laboratory Reports.

8. Harry George's glucose level is _____. The normal range for blood glucose

   is _____.

➡ • Scroll through the Chemistry section of the Laboratory Reports to find the albumin results.

9. Albumin is one measure of nutritional status of the body. Harry George's albumin level was

   _____. The normal range for albumin is _____.

➡ • Click on **Return to Nurses' Station** and then on **MAR**. Choose tab **401** for Harry George's MAR.

10. The first medication listed on Harry George's MAR is _____. This is an antibiotic, and it has a narrow therapeutic range. Peak and trough levels are ordered to track the amount of drug in Harry George's bloodstream.

➡ • Click on **Return to Nurses' Station**; then click on the **Drug** icon in the lower left corner.
   • Use the scroll button to find gentamicin in the drug listings. Read the information and note the therapeutic range for the peak and trough drug levels.
   • Click on **Return to Nurses' Station** and then on **Chart**. Open the chart for **401** and click again on **Laboratory Reports**. Scroll down to the Drug Monitoring section of the reports.

11. Harry George's peak gentamicin level is _____. The trough level is

   _____. Normal therapeutic peak range for gentamicin is

   _____, and normal therapeutic trough range is _____.

   Toxicity occurs at a peak level greater than _____.

Exercise 2

CD-ROM Activity—Diagnostic Tests and Other Laboratory Tests

45 minutes

   • Sign in to work at Pacific View Regional Hospital on the Medical-Surgical Floor for Period of Care 3. (*Note:* If you are already in the virtual hospital from a previous exercise, click on **Leave the Floor** and then **Restart the Program** to get to the sign-in window.)
   • From the Patient List, select Piya Jordan (Room 403).
   • Click on **Go to Nurses' Station** and then on **403**.
   • Read the **Initial Observations**.
   • Click on **Chart** and then on **403**. Click on **Physician's Orders**.
   • Read the orders, noting the laboratory and diagnostic tests that were ordered for Piya Jordan.

Piya Jordan was admitted with abdominal pain, and her diagnostic workup included several tests.

1. Match each test name listed below with its appropriate type of test. (*Note:* Some letters will be used more than once.)

Test Name	Type of Test
_____ CT abdomen	a. Blood chemistry
_____ Urinalysis	b. Blood hematology
_____ Hemoglobin and hematocrit	c. Urine test
_____ KUB and upright	d. Computer enhanced x-ray
_____ Chem 7	e. X-ray
_____ PT/INR	f. Blood clotting study
_____ Chest PA & Lat	g. Blood drug monitoring
_____ Digoxin level	h. Blood serology test
_____ Liver function	
_____ Blood type and crossmatch (T & C)	

2. What does a computed tomography scan show?

3. A KUB is an _____ that shows the _____.

➤ • Click on the **Diagnostic Reports** and read through the reports.

4. On the report of the CT of the abdomen, what was the impression of the radiologist?

5. The chest x-ray report for Piya Jordan was:
   a. normal.
   b. abnormal.

➤ • Click on the **Laboratory Reports** and review.

6. The current value for hemoglobin is _____.

   The current value for hematocrit is _____.

   The normal range for hemoglobin is _____.

   The normal range for hematocrit is _____.

   Piya Jordan is _____.

→ • Click on **Return to Room 403** and then on **MAR**. Select tab **403**. Note the digoxin order.
  • Again, click on **Return to Room 403** and then on the **Drug** icon in the lower left corner. Scroll to find digoxin and read about this drug. Note the therapeutic range.

7. Piya Jordan has atrial fibrillation, which is being treated with digoxin. Digoxin has a narrow

   therapeutic range. The dose of digoxin ordered for Piya Jordan is _____ to be

   given daily. Her digoxin level is _____. The therapeutic range for digoxin is

   _____. Piya Jordan has a _____ level of digoxin
   in her body.

→ • Once again, click on **Return to Room 403** and then on **Chart**.
  • Choose **403** and click on **Laboratory Reports**.
  • Scroll to the Chemistry section and find the potassium level.

8. Piya Jordan's potassium level is _____. The normal range for potassium is

   _____.

→ • Click on **Return to Room 403** and then on **MAR**. Select **403**.

9. How much potassium is Piya Jordan receiving?

  • Click on **Return to Room 403**.
  • Click on **Chart** and then on **403**.
  • Select the **Laboratory Reports** and scroll down to the Special Tests section.

10. Piya Jordan's blood type is _____.

Nutrition, Fluid, and Electrolytes

 Reading Assignment: Fluid, Electrolyte, and Acid-Base Balance (Chapter 25)
Concepts of Basic Nutrition and Cultural Considerations
(Chapter 26)
Diet Therapy and Assisted Feeding (Chapter 27)

Patients: Piya Jordan, Medical-Surgical Floor, Room 403
Pablo Rodriguez, Medical-Surgical Floor, Room 405

Objectives:

1. Identify nutritional components needed for healing.
2. Choose appropriate foods for basic therapeutic diets.
3. Perform teaching for various therapeutic/restricted diets.
4. Recognize abnormal electrolyte values.
5. Recognize risks of selected electrolyte imbalances.

Exercise 1

 CD-ROM Activity—Individual Nutritional Needs

30 minutes

- Sign in to work at Pacific View Regional Hospital on the Medical-Surgical Floor for Period of Care 3. (*Note:* If you are already in the virtual hospital from a previous exercise, click on **Leave the Floor** and then **Restart the Program** to get to the sign-in window.)
- From the Patient List, select Piya Jordan (Room 403).
- Click on **Go to Nurses' Station**.
- Click on **Chart** and then on **403**.
- Review the **History and Physical**.

 1. In the last lesson you determined that Piya Jordan is anemic. She is NPO at present, but when eating again, she will need dietary counseling. She has just had major surgery, and healing should be promoted. When healing from surgery or a major wound, the body needs

more _____. (*Hint:* See page 462 in your textbook.)

2. Vitamin B_{12} can assist with hemoglobin synthesis. Which of the following menu selections will be beneficial to Piya Jordan once she resumes dietary intake?
   a. Citrus fruits
   b. Tomatoes
   c. Eggs
   d. Leafy vegetables

3. Piya Jordan suffers from a form of Kwashiorkor disease.
   a. True
   b. False

4. High-protein diets are beneficial for all individuals.
   a. True
   b. False

5. Vitamin _____ plays a vital role in healing and should be increased in Piya Jordan's diet once she is eating? (*Hint:* See Table 26-4 in your textbook.)

6. Which of the following data are essential when assessing nutritional status? Select all that apply.

   _____ Age

   _____ Hours of sleep per night

   _____ Height

   _____ Occupation

   _____ Income level

   _____ Number of family members

   _____ Usual diet

   _____ Activity

   _____ Food preferences

   _____ General appearance

   _____ Weight gain or loss

   _____ Weight

   _____ Religion

• Click on and review the **Nursing Admission**.

7. Piya Jordan's weight is _____, and her height is _____.

8. What is Piya Jordan's BMI? Considering her height and weight, is her BMI within the acceptable range?

→ • Click on **Return to Nurses' Station** and then on **Kardex**.

• Select tab **403** and scroll to review the Fluid/Nutrition section of the Kardex.

• Next, review the Elimination section of the Kardex.

9. What is Piya Jordan's current diet order? What nutrition is she receiving?

10. Piya Jordan has a nasogastric tube in place. What are the potential functions of a nasogastric tube?

11. The physician has ordered the nasogastric tube be connected to low intermittent suction. What is the underlying rationale of this order? (*Hint:* Refer to Skill 27-1 on page 484-485 in your textbook.)

12. Earlier, you identified a vitamin that Piya Jordan needs to increase in her diet to aid in healing. She will also need additional iron to combat her anemia. Match each of the following foods with the nutrient(s) they will supply.

Food	**Nutrient(s) Supplied**
_____ Orange juice	a. Vitamin C
_____ Red meat	b. Iron
_____ Strawberries	c. Vitamin C and iron
_____ Legumes	
_____ Tomatoes	
_____ Green peppers	
_____ Potatoes	
_____ Whole grains	
_____ Green leafy vegetables	
_____ Fortified cereals	
_____ Grapefruit	

13. Piya Jordan will also need to have sufficient potassium in her diet. Because of her multiple nutrition needs, foods that supply two or more of her needed nutrients are especially valuable in her diet. Match the following foods with the nutrient(s) they supply.

Food	Nutrient(s) Supplied
_____ Bananas	a. Potassium
_____ Oranges	b. Potassium and vitamin C
_____ Broccoli	c. Potassium, vitamin C, and iron
_____ Carrots	d. Potassium and iron
_____ Potatoes	
_____ Meat	
_____ Legumes	
_____ Coffee	

14. After surgery, most patients begin eating with a _____ diet and then progress until they are eating normally again.

Exercise 2

CD-ROM Activity—Fluid and Electrolyte Imbalance

30 minutes

• Sign in to work at Pacific View Regional Hospital on the Medical-Surgical Floor for Period of Care 3. (*Note:* If you are already in the virtual hospital from a previous exercise, click on **Leave the Floor** and then **Restart the Program** to get to the sign-in window.)
• From the Patient List, select Pablo Rodriguez (Room 405).
• Click on **Get Report** and read the report.

1. What two factors mentioned in the shift report are likely to interfere with Pablo Rodriguez's nutritional intake?

2. When preparing to evaluate Pablo Rodriguez's skin turgor, which of the following sites may be used? Select all that apply.

_____ The abdomen

_____ The cheeks

_____ The thigh

_____ The forearm

_____ The palms of the hands

→ • Click on **Go to Nurses' Station** and then on **Chart**.
  • Select **405** and click on **Emergency Department**. Read the entire section.

3. What two fluid and electrolyte problems did Pablo Rodriguez have when admitted to the Emergency Department?

4. Which of the following are signs of dehydration? Select all that apply. (*Hint:* See Box 25-1 on page 440 in your textbook.)

_____ Elevated temperature

_____ Elevated blood pressure

_____ Decreased urine output

_____ Increased pulse rate

_____ Vomiting

_____ Postural hypotension

_____ Thick saliva

_____ Poor skin turgor

5. What signs of dehydration does Pablo Rodriguez exhibit in the Emergency Department?

→ • Click on **Laboratory Reports**. Scroll down to the Chemistry section and find the electrolyte values.

6. Record Pablo Rodriguez's electrolyte values for the days specified in the table below. Indicate whether each value is normal or abnormal.

	Tues	Normal/Abnormal?	Wed	Normal/Abnormal?
Sodium				
Potassium				
Calcium				
Phosphate				
Magnesium				

Read in your medical-surgical textbook about carcinoma of the lung. Note where this type of tumor is likely to metastasize.

→ • Click on the **History and Physical** and review.

7. What risk factor does Pablo Rodriguez have for hypercalcemia?

8. What two signs and symptoms of hypercalcemia does Pablo Rodriguez display?

9. If Pablo Rodriguez's calcium level continues to rise, he will be at risk for life-threatening

   _____.

10. How is Pablo Rodriguez's fluid imbalance treated in the Emergency Department?

It is important to treat Pablo Rodriguez's nausea and vomiting so that he can take in adequate nutrition and stabilize his fluid and electrolytes.

→ • Click on **Physician's Orders** and note the first medication ordered. Scroll down and note the drug ordered for nausea on Tuesday. Read all of the orders.
   • Click on **Return to Nurses' Station** and then click on the **Drug** icon in the lower left corner. Read about these two drugs, which work differently.

11. The drug ordered for Pablo Rodriguez on Wednesday is _____.

    On Tuesday, the drug ordered for nausea was _____.

12. Why do you think Neutra-Phos was ordered for Pablo Rodriguez?

13. The diet the physician ordered for Pablo Rodriguez was _____.

14. Which of the following foods would be allowed on this diet? Select all that apply.

_____ Whole milk

_____ Lean meat

_____ Cheese enchiladas

_____ Fish

_____ Ice cream

_____ Butter

_____ Margarine

_____ Chili beans

_____ Plain vegetables

Exercise 3

CD-ROM Activity—Calculating and Evaluating Intake and Output

15 minutes

- Sign in to work at Pacific View Regional Hospital on the Medical-Surgical Floor for Period of Care 3. (*Note:* If you are already in the virtual hospital from a previous exercise, click on **Leave the Floor** and then **Restart the Program** to get to the sign-in window.)
- From the Patient List, select Pablo Rodriguez (Room 405).
- Click on **Go to Nurses' Station**.
- Click on **EPR** and then on **Login**.
- Choose **405** as the Patient **Intake and Output** as the Category.
- Scroll back to the Wednesday 0700 I&O results.

1. The shift intake for Pablo Rodriguez is _____ mL. His output was _____ mL.

2. Do you think that this indicates he is rehydrating? Explain.

- Using the scroll buttons, note the I&O amounts from 0700 to the current time.

3. Record the patient's I&O amounts below.

Intake

Output

4. Is there still a positive intake balance, indicating rehydration?

5. How many hours ago did Pablo Rodriguez last experience vomiting (emesis)?

6. Which of the following items could you offer Pablo Rodriguez to help rehydrate him? Consider his ordered diet and his post-nausea status. Select all that apply.

_____ Popsicle

_____ Soft-boiled egg

_____ Nonfat milk

_____ Juice (clear)

_____ Boullion

_____ Milkshake

_____ Soft drink

_____ Gelatin

_____ Sherbet

LESSON 14

Promoting Respiration and Oxygenation

 Reading Assignment: Fluid, Electrolyte, and Acid-Base Balance (Chapter 25)
Assisting with Respiration and Oxygen Delivery (Chapter 28)

Patients: Jacquline Catanazaro, Medical-Surgical Floor, Room 402
Patricia Newman, Medical-Surgical Floor, Room 406

Objectives:

1. Recognize abnormalities in SpO_2 and other vital signs that indicate a respiratory problem.
2. Analyze trends in respiratory data.
3. Identify signs of hypoxia.
4. Safely administer oxygen.
5. State the purpose of various respiratory drugs.
6. Assist the patient with respiratory treatments.

Exercise 1

 CD-ROM Activity—Respiratory Assessment

30 minutes

- Sign in to work at Pacific View Regional Hospital on the Medical-Surgical Floor for Period of Care 1. (*Note:* If you are already in the virtual hospital from a previous exercise, click on **Leave the Floor** and then **Restart the Program** to get to the sign-in window.)
- From the Patient List, select Jacquline Catanazaro (Room 402).
- Click on **Get Report** for Jacquline Catanazaro and read the report.
- Click on **Go to Nurses' Station**.
- Click on **Chart** and then on **402**.
- Click on and review the **History and Physical** and **Nursing Admission**.

1. What are Jacquline Catanazaro's medical diagnoses?

2. Which of the following risk factors for the development of respiratory illness are present for Jacquline Catanazaro? Select all that apply.

_____ Age

_____ History of travel

_____ Occupational exposures

_____ Smoking

_____ Family history

_____ Inactivity

_____ Mental illness

→ • Click on **Return to Nurses' Station**.
  • Click on **402** to enter the patient's room.
  • Read the **Initial Observations** and **Clinical Alerts**.
  • Click on **Patient Care** and proceed with a brief, focused respiratory assessment. First, click on **Chest** and then select subcategories **Respiratory** and **Musculoskeletal** in turn (green boxes).

3. Below, record your findings from Pablo Rodriguez's chest assessment.

Respiratory

Musculoskeletal

4. Is Jacquline Catanazaro's SpO_2 within normal limits? (*Hint:* See Skill 28-1 on page 513 in your textbook.)

5. The pulse oximeter is a reading of:
   a. the level of the blood's hematocrit level.
   b. the oxygen saturation of hemoglobin in the blood.
   c. the body's level of $PaCO_2$.
   d. the body's acid-base balance.

6. Jacquline Catanazaro has bilateral wheezes. Which of the following best describes wheezing?
   a. High-pitched, whistling sounds
   b. Deep, snore sounds
   c. Rough, rubbing sounds
   d. Moist, popping sounds

Read in your medical-surgical textbook about asthma, its signs and symptoms, triggering factors, and treatment.

• Click on **Take Vital Signs** and note the respiratory rate.

7. Jacquline Catanazaro's respiratory rate is _____. The normal adult respiratory rate is

   _____.

• Click on **Patient Care** and then on **Nurse-Client Interactions**.
• Select and view the video titled **0730: Intervention—Airway**. (*Note:* Check the virtual clock to see whether enough time has elapsed. You can use the fast-forward feature to advance the time by 2-minute intervals if the video is not yet available. Then click again on **Patient Care** and **Nurse-Client Interactions** to refresh the screen.)

8. During the respiratory crisis being experienced by Jacquline Catanazaro, what is the priority nursing diagnosis?
   a. Activity intolerance
   b. Anxiety
   c. Impaired gas exchange
   d. Ineffective health maintenance

9. What does the nurse tell Jacquline Catanazaro is the current plan?

• Click on **Chart** and then on **402**. Select the **Laboratory Reports** tab. Scroll down to the Arterial Blood Gas section.

10. In the table below, record Jacquline Catanazaro's arterial blood gas results for the times specified.

ABGs	Mon 1030	Wed 0730
PaO_2		
O_2 sat		
$PaCO_2$		
pH		

11. Based on the blood gas values from question 10, what is Jacquline Catanazaro's acid-base abnormality?

Exercise 2

 CD-ROM Activity—Respiratory Treatments

 15 minutes

- Sign in to work at Pacific View Regional Hospital on the Medical-Surgical Floor for Period of Care 1. (*Note:* If you are already in the virtual hospital from a previous exercise, click on **Leave the Floor** and then **Restart the Program** to get to the sign-in window.)
- From the Patient List, select Jacquline Catanazaro (Room 402).
- Click on **Get Report** for Jacquline Catanazaro and read the report.
- Click on **Go to Nurses' Station** and then on **Chart**.
- Select **402**. Click on **Physician's Orders** and read the most current orders.

1. What is the purpose of the nebulizer treatment that is ordered for Jacquline Catanazaro? What medication is ordered?

→ • Click on **Return to Nurses' Station**. Then click on the **Drug** icon in the lower left corner. Scroll to the drug ordered for the nebulizer treatment and read about it.

2. The normal adult dosage for a nebulizer treatment of this medication is _____ mg.

3. This drug has many side effects. Which problems that Jacquline Catanazaro is already displaying might be exacerbated by this drug? Select all that apply.

_____ Stuffy head

_____ Chest tightness

_____ Nervousness

_____ Headache

_____ Tachypnea

_____ Restlessness

→ • Click on **Return to Nurses' Station** and then on **MAR**. Select tab **402** and find the three drugs Jacquline Catanazaro is to receive by inhaler (puffs or MDI). Record these drugs in the table in question 4.

- Once again, click on **Return to Nurses' Station** and then on the **Drug** icon. Find each of the three drugs you listed in the table below. As you read about each drug, record its purpose in the table in question 4.

4. In the table below, identify the three drugs Jacquline Catanazaro is to receive by inhaler. List the purpose of each of these drugs as well.

Inhaler Medication	Purpose

 • You should have noticed in the MAR that Jacquline Catanazaro is also receiving prednisone. Read about this drug in the Drug Guide.

5. How do you think that prednisone helps a person with asthma?

Exercise 3

 CD-ROM Activity—Oxygen Therapy

 30 minutes

- Sign in to work at Pacific View Regional Hospital on the Medical-Surgical Floor for Period of Care 1. (*Note:* If you are already in the virtual hospital from a previous exercise, click on **Leave the Floor** and then **Restart the Program** to get to the sign-in window.)
- From the Patient List, select Patricia Newman (Room 406).
- Click on **Get Report** and read the report.
- Click on **Go to Nurses' Station** and then on **Chart.**
- Click on the chart for **406** and then on the **Physician's Orders**. Read the orders.

1. The physician has ordered oxygen at a rate of _____ by nasal cannula for

   Patricia Newman. The normal range for oxygen flow is _____.

2. An oxygen flow rate of 2 liters/min by nasal cannula provides the patient with

    _____% oxygen.

3. Although Patricia Newman's oxygen saturation is only 88%, the nurse does not increase the flow. Why is it unwise to increase the flow for this patient? (*Hint:* See the History and Physical to read about any long-standing disorders she has. Also see page 521 in your textbook.)

4. Which of the following nursing actions are appropriate when a patient has oxygen ordered by nasal cannula? Select all that apply.

    _____ Check nares to see that they are unobstructed.

    _____ Observe for excoriation on the nose.

    _____ Humidification is required if the flow rate is greater than 2 liters/min.

    _____ Humidification is always required when an O_2 cannula is used.

    _____ Cleanse the nares each shift and check for signs of irritation.

    _____ The cannula may be removed to make eating meals easier.

    _____ Check the oxygen flow rate each time the room is entered to be certain it is set properly.

    _____ Check the back of the ears and lobes for signs of irritation each shift.

5. When a patient has oxygen ordered, safety measures must be instituted. What two things must the nurse do when instituting oxygen therapy?

→ • Still in the chart, click on **Diagnostic Reports** and read the chest x-ray report.

6. What does the impression note on the chest x-ray report say?

7. All patients with a respiratory ailment must be watched for signs of hypoxia. Which of the following is frequently the earliest sign of hypoxia?
   a. Constant cough
   b. Stridor
   c. Substernal retractions
   d. Restlessness

8. Hypoxia and respiratory insufficiency cause different signs and symptoms, depending on how long the patient has been hypoxic. Match each stage of hypoxia with the signs or symptoms common during that period.

Sign or Symptom	**Stage of Hypoxia**
_____ Cyanosis	a. Early
_____ Anxiety	b. Late
_____ Tachypnea	c. Latest
_____ Drop in blood pressure	
_____ Confusion	
_____ Muscle retractions	
_____ Stridor	
_____ Sitting up to breathe	
_____ Dysrhythmia	

9. In a person with emphysema, ineffective coughing spasms may lead to _____

   of the alveoli and may precipitate _____ of the airways.

10. Patricia Newman has pneumonia and a productive cough. She must cough effectively in order to clear her lungs of secretions. What type of coughing would you institute with her?

LESSON ─── 15 ────────────────────────────────

Promoting Urinary and Bowel Elimination

───

Reading Assignment: Promoting Urinary Elimination (Chapter 29)
Promoting Bowel Elimination (Chapter 30)

Patients: Harry George, Medical-Surgical Floor, Room 401
Piya Jordan, Medical-Surgical Floor, Room 403
Pablo Rodriguez, Medical-Surgical Floor, Room 405

Objectives:

1. Identify factors in patient scenarios that interfere with normal urination.
2. Adequately assess elimination status of patients.
3. Recognize abnormal laboratory values for urine tests.
4. Describe proper urinary catheter care.
5. Describe factors that influence bowel elimination for patients.
6. List specific factors that contribute to elimination problems in patients.

Exercise 1

 CD-ROM Activity—Urinary Catheter Care

 30 minutes

- Sign in to work at Pacific View Regional Hospital on the Medical-Surgical Floor for Period of Care 1. (*Note:* If you are already in the virtual hospital from a previous exercise, click on **Leave the Floor** and then **Restart the Program** to get to the sign-in window.)
- From the Patient List, select Piya Jordan (Room 403).
- Click on **Get Report** and review.
- Click on **Go to Nurses' Station**.

Piya Jordan is recovering from a colectomy. She has a Foley catheter in place, and as her nurse, you will be providing appropriate urinary catheter care.

1. Each time you enter Piya Jordan's room, you should check her urinary status by doing which of the following? Select all that apply.

_____ Check the urine in the bag for cloudiness.

_____ Switch the collection bag to the opposite side of the bed.

_____ Verify that the patient is not lying on the catheter.

_____ Irrigate the catheter.

_____ Check the connecting tubing to see that it is hanging straight to the collection bag.

_____ Make certain that urine is flowing into the bag.

_____ Do not raise the collection bag higher than the level of the bladder.

Because Piya Jordan is spending most of her time in bed, and because she has an indwelling catheter, she is at risk for a urinary tract infection. In order to assess her urinary status post-operatively, you need to know her preoperative urinalysis results.

→ • Click on **Chart** and then on **403**. Select **Laboratory Reports**.
• Scroll to the urinalysis results and record them in the table in question 2.

2. Record Piya Jordan's urinalysis results below. In the right column, mark any abnormal results with an X.

Test	Piya Jordan's Results	Abnormal? (X)
Color		
Clarity		
Glucose		
Bilirubin		
Ketones		
Specific gravity		
Blood (occult)		
pH		
Protein		
Nitrite		
Micro: WBC		
RBC		
Bacteria		

It appears that Piya Jordan had a urinary tract infection before surgery. She was also dehydrated from vomiting, which can affect the test results. There was no time to treat the infection before her surgery, so the physician has ordered another urinalysis today.

3. To obtain a urine specimen from a patient with an indwelling catheter, you would clamp the

   catheter _____ the aspiration port for at least _____ minutes before obtaining the specimen.

4. You should use a _____-gauge sterile needle and syringe to obtain the urine specimen from the aspiration port.

5. Aspirate _____ mL of urine for the urine specimen.

6. Below are the steps for obtaining a urine specimen. Number the steps in the correct order.

Steps of the Procedure	Order of Steps
_____ Put on gloves.	a. 1
_____ Open the sterile container.	b. 2
_____ Label the sterile container.	c. 3
_____ Check the order.	d. 4
_____ Clamp off the catheter.	e. 5
_____ Empty the syringe into the sterile container.	f. 6
_____ Aspirate the urine from the catheter.	g. 7
_____ Swab the aspiration port with alcohol.	h. 8
_____ Insert the needle into the aspiration port.	i. 9
_____ Instruct the patient about the procedure.	j. 10
_____ Close the sterile container.	k. 11
_____ Remove and dispose of the gloves.	l. 12

7. Changes can occur in urine if it sits at room temperature for very long. If a urine specimen

   cannot be taken to the laboratory immediately, it should be _____.
   It is best to send the labeled specimen, packaged in a biohazard bag, to the laboratory immediately.

8. Piya Jordan is at risk for bladder infection for a variety of reasons. Which of the following apply? Select all that apply.

   _____ Urinary stasis from bed rest and inactivity

   _____ Bowel colectomy

   _____ Dehydration from nausea and vomiting before surgery

_____ NPO status with intravenous fluid administration

_____ Presence of an indwelling catheter

_____ Obesity

_____ Decreased bladder tone and possible incomplete emptying due to age

9. What is the single most important nursing measure to prevent infection for the patient who has an indwelling catheter? (*Hint:* Use critical thinking for this question.)

10. What signs and symptoms would you look for that might tell you your patient is experiencing a bladder infection (cystitis)?

11. People who are prone to recurrent bladder infections should drink plenty of water (2500-3000 mL a day) and should void at least every _____ hours.

12. When caring for Piya Jordan, the nurse must know that the hourly urine output should be at least:
    a. 25 mL
    b. 30 mL
    c. 35 mL
    d. 45 mL

→ • Click on **Return to Nurses' Station.**
   • Click on **EPR** and **Login**.
   • Select **403** as the Patient and **Intake and Output** as the Category.
   • Review the urinary elimination patterns for Piya Jordan.

13. Piya Jordan has a urinary output that, when averaged, meets the minimum hourly amount.
    a. True
    b. False

Exercise 2

CD-ROM Activity—Assisting with Bowel Elimination

30 minutes

• Sign in to work at Pacific View Regional Hospital on the Medical-Surgical Floor for Period of Care 1. (*Note:* If you are already in the virtual hospital from a previous exercise, click on **Leave the Floor** and then **Restart the Program** to get to the sign-in window.)
• From the Patient List, select Pablo Rodriguez (Room 405).

- Click on **Get Report** and review the report.
- Click on **Go to Nurses' Station**.
- Click on **405** to visit Pablo Rodriguez.
- Read the **Initial Observations**.
- Click on **MAR** and go to the page for Pablo Rodriguez (**405**).

1. What medication is Pablo Rodriguez receiving that can cause constipation?

2. Refer to the preceding question. What impact does the medication have on bowel elimination?
   a. Slows peristalsis
   b. Draws water from stool in the lower colon
   c. Reduces neurologic stimuli related to the urge to defecate
   d. Slows the digestive processes in the stomach

→ - Click on **Return to Room 405**.
- Click on **Patient Care** and perform an abdominal assessment on Pablo Rodriguez. Record your findings in the chart below.

3. Record your findings from Pablo Rodriguez's abdominal assessment below.

Integumentary

Musculoskeletal

Gastrointestinal

→ - Click on **EPR** and on **Login**. Choose **405** from the Patient menu. From the Category menu, select **Gastrointestinal**. Enter your findings from the abdominal assessment in the correct EPR columns using the symbols listed for each line.

4. When did Pablo Rodriguez have his last bowel movement? What were the characteristics of his stool? (*Hint:* See earlier entries in the EPR.)

5. Why do you think Pablo Rodriguez is at risk for constipation and fecal impaction?

6. The physician has ordered a mineral oil enema. When giving a mineral oil enema, you know

that it should be retained for _____ in order to be effective.

→ • Click on **Exit EPR** and then on **MAR**. (Again, be sure you are looking at the correct page for Pablo Rodriguez!) Note the medications on the MAR that are used to prevent or treat constipation. Click on the **Drug** icon in the lower left corner to look up any medications with which you are unfamiliar.

7. Below, list the medications from Pablo Rodriguez's MAR that treat or prevent constipation. For each medication, list the action and/or use.

Medication	Action/Use

8. If the physician orders a soap suds enema for Pablo Rodriguez, there are specific steps to be followed.

a. How would you position Pablo Rodriguez to administer the enema?

b. During a soap suds enema, how should the container be positioned?

c. What is the rationale for running the solution into the patient's body slowly?

d. What should be the temperature of the solution?

Exercise 3

 CD-ROM Activity—Measures to Prevent Constipation

30 minutes

- Sign in to work at Pacific View Regional Hospital on the Medical-Surgical Floor for Period of Care 2. (*Note:* If you are already in the virtual hospital from a previous exercise, click on **Leave the Floor** and then **Restart the Program** to get to the sign-in window.)
- From the Patient List, select Harry George (Room 401).
- Click on **Get Report** and review the report.
- Click on **Go to Nurses' Station**.
- Click on **Kardex** and then on tab **401**. Check what type of activity is ordered for Harry George.
- Click on **Return to Nurses' Station** and then on **Chart**. Click on **401** and then on **Nurse's Notes**. Read about Harry George's food intake.
- Click on **Return to Nurses' Station** and then on **MAR**. Select tab **401** and note the medications Harry George is taking that could contribute to constipation. (*Hint:* What pain medication is he receiving?)

  1. How has Harry George been eating? What factors in his eating pattern could contribute to constipation?

→ • Once again, click on **Return to Nurses' Station** and then on **Chart**. Select the **Expired MARs** and read through them.

  2. It appears that Harry George is receiving the pain medication _____

     _____ about every _____. He has had _____ doses since admission. (*Hint:* Remember to check today's MAR also.)

→ • Click on **Nursing Admission** and review the Elimination section.

  3. Harry George's usual bowel pattern is to have a bowel movement _____.

→ • Click on **Return to Nurses' Station** and click on **EPR**. Select **401** as the Patient and **Gastrointestinal** as the Category. Use the arrows to scroll back to see when Harry George had a bowel movement.

4. Harry George's last bowel movement was _____.

   He _____ (does/does not) appear to be constipated.

5. Often bisacodyl suppositories are ordered prn in case the patient becomes constipated. How does this suppository work?

6. When administering a bisacodyl suppository, you instruct the patient to try to retain it for at

   least _____.

7. Many actions can help prevent elimination problems. For each action listed below, indicate whether the action can help prevent constipation (mark with "a"), help prevent urinary tract infection (mark with "b"), or help prevent both problems (mark with "c").

Action	Elimination Problem It Helps Prevent
_____ Increase fluids to 2500-3000 mL per day	a. Constipation
_____ Increase fresh fruits and vegetables in the diet	b. Urinary tract infection
_____ Exercise every day	c. Constipation and urinary tract infection
_____ Cleanse the perineum from front to back	
_____ Increase vitamin C intake	
_____ Empty the bladder after intercourse	
_____ Pay attention to the urge to defecate	
_____ Use aid such as hot coffee, hot water, and lemon juice	
_____ Avoid citrus fruits and juices	
_____ Wear cotton underwear	

Preparation for Drug Administration

 Reading Assignment: Pharmacology and Preparation for Drug Administration
(Chapter 33)
Administering Oral, Topical, and Inhalant Medications
(Chapter 34)

Patients: Harry George, Medical-Surgical Floor, Room 401
Jacquline Catanazaro, Medical-Surgical Floor, Room 402

Objectives:

1. Give the rationale for why a patient is receiving a particular drug.
2. Calculate drug dosages accurately.
3. Identify the nursing implications for drugs a patient is to receive.
4. Describe the correct steps for administration of medications.

Exercise 1

 CD-ROM Activity—Medication Knowledge

30 minutes

• Sign in to work at Pacific View Regional Hospital on the Medical-Surgical Floor for Period of Care 1. (*Note:* If you are already in the virtual hospital from a previous exercise, click on **Leave the Floor** and then **Restart the Program** to get to the sign-in window.)
• From the Patient List, select Jacquline Catanazaro (Room 402).
• Click on **Get Report** and read the report.
• Click on **Go to Nurses' Station**.
• Click on **Chart** and then on **402**. Select **History and Physical** and review.

1. According to the History and Physical, what diagnoses/problems does Jacquline Catanazaro have?

• Click on **Return to Nurses' Station**, and then on **MAR**. Select tab **402** and find the medications requested in question 2 below.

• Again, click on **Return to Nurses' Station**. To complete question 2, consult the Drug Guide by clicking on the **Drug** icon in the lower left corner of your screen.

2. List the oral and topical medications ordered on Jacquline Catanazaro's MAR. For each medication, provide the reason she is receiving it.

Medication	Reason for Receiving Medication

3. Match each medication Jacquline Catanazaro is receiving with its classification or mechanism of action.

Medication	Classification/Mechanism of Action
_____ Prednisone	a. Antipsychotic/antidepressant
_____ Amoxicillin	b. Nonsteroidal antiinflammatory
_____ Ziprasidone	c. Antipsychotic
_____ Ibuprofen	d. Antibiotic
_____ Albuterol	e. Corticosteroid/systemic
_____ Beclomethasone	f. Bronchodilator/antiasthmatic
_____ Ipratropium bromide	g. Adrenocorticosteroid/antiinflammatory
	h. Anticholinergic/bronchodilator

4. Number the following steps for medication administration in the correct order.

Medication Administration Step	Order of Steps
_____ Check that this is the correct date and time the medication is ordered.	a. Step 1
	b. Step 2
_____ Check each medication against the MAR, comparing drug name, dose, and route as you pull it from the patient's drawer, bin, or automatic dispenser machine.	c. Step 3
	d. Step 4
_____ Verify that today's date is before the expiration of each medication.	e. Step 5
_____ Wash your hands.	f. Step 6
_____ Perform a second check of the medication for right drug, dose, time, and route.	g. Step 7
	h. Step 8
_____ Initial the MAR for each dose of medication administered.	i. Step 9
_____ Go to the patient.	j. Step 10
_____ Open the medication.	k. Step 11
_____ Verify the patient's identification by checking his or her armband against the name and number on the MAR and asking the patient to state his or her name.	
_____ Recheck each medication against the MAR for the right drug, dose, route, and time.	
_____ Administer the medications.	

➤ • Return to the listing in the Drug Guide for prednisone.

5. Prednisone acts by:
   a. preventing release of corticosteroid in the body.
   b. increasing the release of adrenocorticosteroid.
   c. preventing tissue response to the inflammatory process.
   d. increasing the cell-mediated immune response.

6. Because of this action, prednisone may mask _____.

7. Patients who are receiving prednisone may experience _____ as a side effect, which makes them feel fatigued.

8. A bone disorder that occurs with long-term prednisone use is _____.

9. When a patient is receiving prednisone, the nurse must do appropriate teaching. Which of the following points would you cover in a teaching plan? Select all that apply.

_____ Single daily dose should be taken before 9:00 a.m.

_____ Take it only on an empty stomach, an hour before a meal.

_____ Report any other signs of infection.

_____ It is okay to have an occasional glass of wine while taking prednisone.

_____ Caffeine intake should be limited.

_____ Report weight loss promptly.

_____ Mood swings are not uncommon.

_____ Do not stop taking the drug abruptly.

10. You will be teaching Jacquline Catanazaro how to properly use her MDI of albuterol. The proper steps are listed below. Number these steps in the proper order.

Step for Using MDI for Albuterol	**Order of Steps**
_____ Wait 1 minute between puffs when more than one puff is ordered.	a. Step 1
_____ Place the mouthpiece 1-2 inches in front of your mouth.	b. Step 2
_____ Sit or stand up to use the inhaler.	c. Step 3
_____ Press the canister down while inhaling.	d. Step 4
_____ Shake the canister several times before beginning.	e. Step 5
_____ Breathe out through your mouth, emptying the lungs.	f. Step 6
_____ Use a bronchodilator MDI before a steroid MDI.	g. Step 7

→ • Scroll to find amoxicillin in the Drug Guide.

11. Are there any drug interactions between amoxicillin and the other drugs Jacquline Catanazaro is taking? If so, what are they?

12. What are the common GI side effects of amoxicillin?

13. For the dose of amoxicillin ordered to be given at 1500, what would you do to try to prevent the GI side effects?

  Exercise 2

 CD-ROM Activity—More Medications

30 minutes

- Sign in to work at Pacific View Regional Hospital on the Medical-Surgical Floor for Period of Care 1. (*Note:* If you are already in the virtual hospital from a previous exercise, click on **Leave the Floor** and then **Restart the Program** to get to the sign-in window.)
- From the Patient List, select Harry George (Room 401).
- Click on **Get Report** and read the report.
- Click on **Go to Nurses' Station**.
- Click on **401** to visit the patient's room.
- Inside the room, click on **Check Allergies**.
- Now click on **Chart** and then on **401**; select the tab for **History and Physical**. Read about Harry George.

1. What are Harry George's diagnoses and/or problems?

→ • Click on **Return to Room 401** and then on the **MAR**; verify that the page is for Harry George.

2. Does Harry George have any allergies to medication?

3. Medication may have a variety of therapeutic effects. Harry George has thiamine 100 mg PO or IM ordered. Which of the following is the most likely rationale for this order in his case?
   a. Reduces anorexia
   b. Increases effectiveness of antibiotic therapy
   c. Promotes carbohydrate metabolism
   d. Reduces ketones in the urine

4. The normal adult dosage of thiamine is up to _____.

   The order for Harry George _____ (is/is not) within the normal dosage range.

5. Are there any criteria that indicate the thiamine should be given IM?

→ • Click on **Return to Room 401**.

   • Click on the **Drug** icon and scroll to gentamicin. Read about this drug.

6. What is the toxic level for gentamicin?

7. There are many nursing implications for gentamicin. Which of the following actions are the most important? Select all that apply.

   _____ Monitor intake and output.

   _____ Administer the drug between meals.

   _____ Ask the patient about ringing in the ears or decreased hearing.

   _____ Administer the drug only with a meal.

   _____ Report nausea promptly.

   _____ Give IM injection quickly.

   _____ Do not give if patient is dehydrated.

   _____ Assess for skin rash.

   _____ Report diarrhea promptly.

8. Are there any drug interactions between gentamicin and the other drugs Harry George is receiving?

9. Harry George has trimethobenzamide HCl 250 mg (Tigan) PO ordered q6h prn nausea and

   vomiting. Trimethobenzamide HCl is a(n) _____ class drug.

10. Harry George is also receiving chlordiazepoxide HCl, and hydromorphone. What is the potential interaction effect of these drugs with trimethobenzamide HCl?

11. Harry George has glyburide ordered to help treat his diabetes. What is the mechanism of action of this drug?

12. What type or class of drug is glyburide?

13. Glyburide begins working within _____ to _____ minutes.

14. The glyburide is listed on the MAR to be given at 0800. What would you want to know before administering the drug at that time?

15. Below, list the PO and topical drugs that are ordered for Harry George. For each drug, provide its action or the reason for administration.

Medication	Action and/or Reason for Administration

Oral Medication Administration

 Reading Assignment: Pharmacology and Preparation for Drug Administration
(Chapter 33)
Administering Oral, Topical, and Inhalant Medications
(Chapter 34)

Patients: Harry George, Medical-Surgical Floor, Room 401
Clarence Hughes, Medical-Surgical Floor, Room 404

Objectives:

1. Safely administer oral medications.
2. Identify the nursing assessments necessary before administering a drug.
3. Know the potential side effects and adverse effects of the drugs being administered.
4. Identify any interactions between drugs being administered and other drugs the patient is taking.

Exercise 1

 CD-ROM Activity—Administering PO Medications

45 minutes

- Sign in to work at Pacific View Regional Hospital on the Medical-Surgical Floor for Period of Care 1. (*Note:* If you are already in the virtual hospital from a previous exercise, click on **Leave the Floor** and then **Restart the Program** to get to the sign-in window.)
- From the Patient List, select Harry George (Room 401).
- Click on **Get Report** and review the information about this patient.
- Click on **Go to Nurses' Station** and then on **401**.
- Click on **Patient Care** and then on **Medication Administration**.
- Prepare to give Harry George his 0800 PO medications. (*Hint:* First click on **MAR** and find his orders.)

    1. Which oral medications is Harry George scheduled to receive at 0800 according to his MAR?

2. Are there any assessments that you need to make before preparing and administering these medications? (*Hint:* Harry George is diabetic, so you might want to know his morning blood glucose determination. Click on **Return to Room 401** and then on **Chart**. Select the chart for **401** and click on **Nurse's Notes**.)

3. Which of the following system assessments should you make before giving the 0800 PO medications? Select all that apply.

_____ Chest

_____ Abdomen

_____ Head & Neck

_____ Upper Extremities

_____ Lower Extremities

_____ Back & Spine

→ • Click on **Return to Room 401**.
   • Now click on **Medication Room** and prepare Harry George's 0800 medications.
   • Click on **Unit Dosage** or on the unit dose cart and then on drawer **401** to access Harry George's medications.
   • Click to highlight the correct drug to be removed from the drawer.
   • Verify the MAR order against the medication information on dosage and route on the unit dose label (shown on the right side of the screen).
   • Click on **Put Medication on Tray**.
   • After each medication has been moved to the tray, click on **Review Your Medications** and again verify the drug, dosage, and route compared against the MAR information. This is your second check of the medication after removing it from the drawer.
   • After your review of each medication, click on **Close Drawer** in the lower right corner of the screen and then click on **View Medication Room**.
   • Now click on **Preparation** or on the tray sitting on the counter on the left side of your screen. Verify the drug label with the order and click **Prepare**. This activates the Preparation Wizard. Supply any requested information; then click **Next**.
   • Click on the correct patient's room number and name and then click on **Finish**.

4. Below, document the medications ordered for Harry George at 0800.

Medication Order	Route	To Be Administered By You?

5. Glyburide can increase the activity of oral _____.

6. Is Harry George receiving the above-mentioned drug?

➡ • Click on **Return to Medication Room** and then on **401**.
   • Inside the patient's room, click on **Check Armband** to correctly identify Harry George as the patient for whom your medications are intended.
   • Now click on **Check Allergies** and review this information.
   • Click on **Patient Care** and then on **Medication Administration**.
   • Click on the down arrow next to **Select**.
   • Click on **Administer**. Choose the correct route from the drop-down menu. Next, select the correct method.
   • Once you are sure everything has been checked three times and that the medication meets the order criteria and the correct time, click on **Administer to Patient**. Document that you have given the drug by clicking on **Yes**. Repeat this process for each medication on your tray. Finally, click **Finish**.

7. What, if any, allergy does Harry George have?

8. Glyburide peaks in _____ hours and lasts _____ hours.

9. Why is it important that Harry George eat his meals when he is taking this medication?

10. Patients with diabetes can become hypoglycemic or hyperglycemic for a variety of reasons. It is important that the nurse know whether this is happening. Below, match each sign or symptom with the correct disorder.

Sign or Symptom

Disorder

_____ Blurred vision

a. Hyperglycemia

_____ Thirst

b. Hypoglycemia

_____ Shakiness or tremors

_____ Rapid respirations

_____ Headache

_____ Tachycardia

_____ Hunger

_____ Cool, clammy skin

_____ Nausea or vomiting

_____ Increased urination

- Click on **Leave the Floor** and then select **Look at Your Preceptor's Evaluation**. Click on **Medication Scorecard** to see how you did with the medication administration for Harry George.

Exercise 2

 CD-ROM Activity—Administering More Medications

 30 minutes

- Sign in to work at Pacific View Regional Hospital on the Medical-Surgical Floor for Period of Care 1. (*Note:* If you are already in the virtual hospital from a previous exercise, click on **Leave the Floor** and then **Restart the Program** to get to the sign-in window.)
- From the Patient List, select Clarence Hughes (Room 404).
- Click on **Get Report** and review the information.
- Click on **Go to Nurses' Station**.
- Click on **MAR** and note the medications to be administered to Clarence Hughes at 0800. (*Hint:* You will need to record these orders in the table in question 2.)
- Click on **Return to Nurses' Station** and then on **404** to go to the patient's room.
- Click on **Clinical Alerts** and determine what assessments need to be made before you administer medications. (*Hint:* You will use this information to answer question 5.)

1. What is the first thing you should do before going to the Medication Room and pulling medications for patients from the drawers or bins?

Check mar and right patient

2. Below, copy the orders for the oral 0800 medications, as well as any prn medications, to be given to Clarence Hughes.

Medication Order	Route	Classification of Medication
Docusate sodium 100mg PO daily	PO	laxative
Celecoxib 100mg PO BID	PO	
enoxaparin 30mg every 12 hours	subQ	
oxycodon		

3. What does a valid medication order contain?

Pt full name
frequency
Route

4. Based on your review of the **Clinical Alerts** what assessments should you perform?

allergy   complaining of pain and allergy

 • Click on **Check Allergies.**

5. Does Clarence Hughes have any drug allergies?

NO

6. Is the order on the MAR for oxycodone with acetaminophen a valid order? If not, what is missing? yes

7. What would you do before giving the oxycodone with acetaminophen?

Call pharm
Drug guide

8. When administering medications to Clarence Hughes, is it is important to be aware of the findings of ___pharmokinetic___ research, which indicates that differing groups may metabolize medications differently.

- Click on **Medication Room** at the bottom of the screen.
- Click on **Unit Dosage** or on the unit dosage cart and then on drawer **404**.
- Click on the first medication you wish to administer to Clarence Hughes at 0800. Verify the unit dose medication label with the order as you take it from the drawer, following the five rights.
- Click on **Put Medication on Tray**. Continue this process for each medication that you are going to administer.
- Click on **Close Drawer** and then on **View Medication Room** in the lower right corner.
- Click on **Automated System** to obtain the controlled drug. Click **Login**.
- Select **Clarence Hughes, 404**. Choose the correct drawer for the medication you want. (Assume the order is for the 5/325 dosage.) Click **Open Drawer**.
- Select the correct medication and click on **Put Medication on Tray**. Then click on **Close Drawer**.
- Click on **Review Your Medications**. Highlight each medication in turn and perform your second medication check with the drug order. Use the Five Rights!
- Click on **Return to Medication Room** and then on **View Medication Room**.

9. What do you need to do before you prepare the medications you have put on the tray?

Check with MAR

- Click on **Preparation** or on the tray on the counter on the left side of the screen.
- Click on **Prepare** and then supply any information requested by the Preparation Wizard before clicking **Finish**. Continue this process for each medication.
- Click on **Return to Medication Room**.
- Click on **404** to return to Clarence Hughes' room.

10. You have just entered Clarence Hughes' room. What should you do at this point?

check arm band
Check med before admin
open before admin

11. When and how do you perform your third check of the medications?

before administered

 • Click on **Patient Care** and then on **Medication Administration**.

• Follow the steps in the Administration Wizard until you have administered all the medications you prepared. (*Hint:* If you need help with any of these steps, refer to the **Getting Started** section of this workbook.)

12. What do you need to do after you have administered all of the medications for this time period?

check in frequently to see if pain level had decreased.

 • Click on **Leave the Floor**.

• Click on **Look at Your Preceptor's Evaluation**. Click on **Medication Scorecard** and review the evaluation.

18 ————————————————

Administering Injections and Topical Medications

————————————————————————————————————

 Reading Assignment: Administering Oral, Topical, and Inhalant Medications
(Chapter 34)
Administering Intradermal, Subcutaneous, and Intramuscular
Injections (Chapter 35)

Patients: Harry George, Medical-Surgical Floor, Room 401
Clarence Hughes, Medical-Surgical Floor, Room 404
Patricia Newman, Medical-Surgical Floor, Room 406

Objectives:

1. Correctly administer subcutaneous injections.
2. Identify injection sites for intramuscular injections.
3. Correctly administer an intramuscular injection.
4. Safely administer ophthalmic medications.
5. Use correct technique when applying a medicated skin patch.

Exercise 1

 CD-ROM Activity—Administering Insulin

🕐 30 minutes

- Sign in to work at Pacific View Regional Hospital on the Medical-Surgical Floor for Period of Care 1. (*Note:* If you are already in the virtual hospital from a previous exercise, click on **Leave the Floor** and then **Restart the Program** to get to the sign-in window.)
- From the Patient List, select Harry George (Room 401).
- Click on **Get Report** and review the information.
- Click on **Go to Nurses' Station**.
- Click on **401** to visit Harry George. Let's assume that when you ask the patient how he is feeling, he tells you that he is a little nauseous.
- Click on **MAR** to see what medication is ordered that may help relieve the nausea.
- Click on **Return to 401** and visit Harry George to see whether he needs anything else before you prepare this medication.

1. Harry George's MAR indicates he is to receive thiamine 100 mg once a day. What is the maximum safe dose for an adult?

 • Click on **Medication Room** and then on **Unit Dosage**. Choose the drawer for **401**.
   • Click on the correct drug to be removed from the drawer.
   • Verify the MAR order with the dosage and route information on the unit dosage label.
   • Click on **Put Medication on Tray**.
   • Perform your second check of the medication by clicking on **Review Your Medications**. Once again, verify the drug, dosage, and route—and that it is intended to be given at this time on this date.
   • Click on **Return to Medication Room**, then on **Close Drawer**, and then on **View Medication Room**.

2. What size syringe and needle will you choose to give this injection to Harry George?

3. What must you do before beginning to prepare the medications?

 • Click on **Preparation** or on the tray on the counter. Verify the drug label against the order and click **Prepare**. Supply any information requested by the Preparation Wizard; then click **Next**.
   • Click on the correct room number; then click **Finish** and **Return to Medication Room**.
   • Click on **401** to return to the patient's room.

4. What should you do when you enter Harry George's room before giving his injection?

5. What precautions should you take when administering this injection?

• Now click on **Patient Care** and then on **Medication Administration**.

- Click on the arrow next to **Select** and choose **Administer**. After the Administration Wizard appears, choose the route, method, and site from the drop-down menus.
- Click on **Administer the Medication** and answer **Yes** to the next question.

6. The other site into which you could inject the thiamine is the _____.

7. Harry George has already had his early morning insulin. You will be giving him insulin before lunch later today. Before giving this next dose of insulin, what would you need to do?

8. When drawing up the indicated amount of insulin, what safety precaution should you take?

9. When both regular and NPH insulin are ordered to be given together, you would draw up

   the _____ insulin first.

10. Regular insulin has its onset in _____, peaks in _____, and has a

    duration of _____.

11. What area is preferred for insulin injection?

Exercise 2

 CD-ROM Activity—Heparin Administration and Ophthalmic Medication Administration

🕐 30 minutes

- Sign in to work at Pacific View Regional Hospital on the Medical-Surgical Floor for Period of Care 1. (*Note:* If you are already in the virtual hospital from a previous exercise, click on **Leave the Floor** and then **Restart the Program** to get to the sign-in window.)
- From the Patient List, select Clarence Hughes (Room 404).
- Click on **Get Report** and review the information.
- Click on **Go to Nurses' Station**.
- Click on **MAR** and check for the enoxaparin injection that Clarence Hughes is to receive.

1. Complete the table below based on the MAR order for enoxaparin.

Drug Order	Classification	Action	Precautions

2. What is the most likely reason enoxaparin is ordered for Clarence Hughes?

3. Enoxaparin is usually given after knee replacement surgery for an average of

   _____.

4. If Clarence Hughes experienced bleeding problems, you would give the antidote for

   enoxaparin, which is _____.

5. When administering enoxaparin, which of the following would you do to provide Clarence Hughes with the dose ordered? Select all that apply.

   _____ Use any subcutaneous site.

   _____ Use the prefilled syringe of 0.3 mL.

   _____ Use a 5/8-inch needle at a 45-degree angle.

   _____ Use a 1/2-inch needle at a 90-degree angle.

   _____ Use a 2-mL syringe.

   _____ Use the abdominal area lateral and below the umbilicus.

   _____ Pull the tissue taut before introducing the needle.

   _____ Pinch up the tissue in a roll before introducing the needle.

   _____ Inject deep into the subcutaneous tissue.

   _____ Do not aspirate before injecting this medication.

   _____ Rub the area gently after injection to hasten absorption.

   _____ Wait at least 15 seconds after injecting before withdrawing the needle.

6. What laboratory test would you want to check to see whether this drug is effective?

 • Return to Clarence Hughes' MAR and note the ophthalmic solutions ordered for him. Read about these medications in the Drug Guide.

7. Timolol and pilocarpine are used for what disorder?

8. If Clarence Hughes does not use his eye drops, what could be the consequences?

9. If these are new medications for Clarence Hughes, what points of patient teaching should you cover? (*Hint:* Check a pharmacology book or nursing drug handbook.)

Exercise 3

 CD-ROM Activity—Transdermal Medication

 15 minutes

• Sign in to work at Pacific View Regional Hospital on the Medical-Surgical Floor for Period of Care 1. (*Note:* If you are already in the virtual hospital from a previous exercise, click on **Leave the Floor** and then **Restart the Program** to get to the sign-in window.)
• From the Patient List, select Patricia Newman (Room 406).
• Click on **Get Report** and review the information.
• Click on **Go to Nurses' Station**.
• Click on **MAR** and then on **406**. Note the transdermal patch ordered for Patricia Newman.

1. Below, list the information for the transdermal patch ordered for Patricia Newman. (*Hint:* Consult a pharmacology book, nursing drug handbook, or the Drug Guide on the CD-ROM.)

Medication Order	Classification	Action/Reason for Administration

2. Was the transdermal skin patch applied on Tuesday? (*Hint:* Go to the chart and check the **Expired MARs** to see whether the drug was administered.)

3. What should you do with the information you just discovered?

4. Where should a skin patch be placed on the body?

5. After application, the patch should be _____ for identification of when it was applied.

6. When applying a new transdermal patch, you should always _____

_____.

7. What is necessary to do to ensure that the transdermal patch will adhere properly?

LESSON 19

Caring for Patients Receiving Intravenous Therapy

 Reading Assignment: Administering Intravenous Solutions and Medications
(Chapter 36)

Patients: Harry George, Medical-Surgical Floor, Room 401
Piya Jordan, Medical-Surgical Floor, Room 403

Objectives:

1. Follow safe practice in the administration of IV fluids.
2. Identify signs of IV infiltration.
3. List the signs and symptoms of complications of IV therapy.
4. Perform assessments essential for the patient receiving IV fluids.
5. Monitor patients for side effects of IV medications.

Exercise 1

 CD-ROM Activity—Monitoring the Patient Receiving Intravenous Therapy

30 minutes

- Sign in to work at Pacific View Regional Hospital on the Medical-Surgical Floor for Period of Care 1. (*Note:* If you are already in the virtual hospital from a previous exercise, click on **Leave the Floor** and then **Restart the Program** to get to the sign-in window.)
- From the Patient List, select Harry George (Room 401).
- Click on **Get Report** and read the report.
- Click on **Go to Nurses' Station** and then click on **Chart**.
- Click on the chart for **401**. Select the tab for **Physician's Orders** and note the solutions and medications Harry George is currently receiving intravenously.

1. Below, list the intravenous solutions and medications ordered for Harry George. For each medication, give the classification, along with its action or the reason it is ordered.

Medication Order	Classification	Action/Reason for Administration

You should become familiar with the side effects and nursing implications for these drugs since you are caring for Harry George.

 2. Name the three most important nursing implications for the benzodiazepine drugs. (*Hint:* Consult a pharmacology book, nursing drug handbook, or the Drug Guide on the CD-ROM.)

➡ • Now click on **Return to Nurses' Station** and then on **401**. Inside the patient's room, click on **Patient Care** and then on **Upper Extremities**. Assess Harry George's IV site.

3. Where is Harry George's IV site located?

4. Document your findings concerning the IV site.

5. What question(s) would you ask Harry George about his IV site?

6. If tubing that delivers 15 drops per mL is being used, the IV will be flowing at _____ drops per minute.

7. What is the purpose of administering an isotonic intravenous solution?

→ • Click on **Chart** and then on **401**. Click on **Nurse's Notes** and review.

8. As far as you can tell, when was Harry George's IV cannula inserted?

9. Is the IV cannula due to be changed today? Are there any indications that it should be changed? (*Hint:* Click on **Emergency Department** and read the ED nurse's notes.)

→ • Click on **Return to Room 401**.
   • Click on **EPR** and **Login**. Select **401** as the Patient and **IV** as the Category. Highlight the data to see the pertinent abbreviations for interpretation of the documentation.

10. How often should Harry George's tubing be changed?
    a. Every 12 to 24 hours
    b. Every 24 hours
    c. Every 24 to 48 hours
    d. Every 72 hours

- When a patient is receiving intravenous fluid, the nurse should monitor the electrolyte values to determine whether the intravenous therapy is causing any electrolyte imbalance.
- Click on **Exit EPR**.
- Click on **Chart** and then **401**. Select **Laboratory Reports**.

11. Harry George's potassium level is _____. His sodium level is _____. His

_____ level is above normal and most likely indicates a state of slight dehydration. The slightly elevated chloride level is consistent with the sodium level.

12. Which of the following laboratory reports would provide the best indication of whether the antibiotics Harry George is receiving are effective?
   a. Urinalysis
   b. Culture and sensitivity
   c. Complete blood cell count
   d. Gentamycin peak and trough levels
   e. Electrolyte panel

Exercise 2

 CD-ROM Activity—Complications of Intravenous Therapy

 15 minutes

1. Match each sign or symptom below with its related IV therapy complication.

Sign or Symptom	Complication of IV Therapy
_____ Coolness surrounding the IV site	a. Infiltration
_____ Redness at the IV site	b. Phlebitis
_____ Sudden drop in BP with increase in pulse rate	c. Thrombophlebitis
_____ Redness of the vein used for IV therapy	d. Infection at site
	e. Air embolus
_____ Red site with itching and rash	f. Speed shock
_____ Hardness along the vein used for IV therapy	g. Infection
_____ Fever, chills, general malaise	h. Circulatory overload
_____ Flushed face and severe headache	i. Allergic reaction to IV medication
_____ Warmth at the IV site	
_____ IV flow sluggish with redness and tenderness at site	
_____ IV site hot, red, and painful	
_____ Elevated BP, dyspnea, crackles in lungs	

2. What should you do if IV infiltration occurs?

3. If the IV flow has slowed considerably after the patient has been up for a sponge bath, what basic actions would you take before assuming that the cannula is clotted?

4. How often should you check on your patient to assess the IV site and flow rate when IV therapy is in progress?

5. You are monitoring your patient's IV. It is to run at 100 mL/hr. The tubing the hospital uses delivers 10 drops per mL. How many drops per minute should the IV deliver?
   a. 16 drops a minute
   b. 21 drops a minute
   c. 28 drops a minute
   d. 25 drops a minute

Exercise 3

 CD-ROM Activity—Monitoring the Patient Receiving a Blood Transfusion

 30 minutes

- Sign in to work at Pacific View Regional Hospital on the Medical-Surgical Floor for Period of Care 2. (*Note:* If you are already in the virtual hospital from a previous exercise, click on **Leave the Floor** and then **Restart the Program** to get to the sign-in window.)
- From the Patient List, select Piya Jordan (Room 403).
- Click on **Get Report** and read the report.
- Click on **Go to Nurses' Station** and then on **Chart**.
- Click on **403** and select the **Physician's Notes**. Review to find out what blood product is planned for Piya Jordan.

1. The physician has planned to give Piya Jordan 2 units of _____.

2. Why is Piya Jordan receiving this blood transfusion? What laboratory parameters would you check before the blood is administered so that you will know later whether the transfusion was effective? (*Hint:* See the Laboratory Reports in her chart.)

3. In order for this blood product to be administered, Piya Jordan should have an

    _____ IV cannula in place.

➡ • Click on the **Nurse's Notes** and read the note for Wednesday at 0745.

4. Is the IV cannula that Piya Jordan has in place the correct size for the blood product transfusion?

5. Is there a valid consent signed by Piya Jordan for the blood transfusion?

6. Which of the following are pertinent guidelines when administering a blood transfusion? Select all that apply.

    _____ Blood must be kept refrigerated until it is administered.

    _____ Gloves must be used when discontinuing a blood product transfusion.

    _____ Blood products are administered along with D_5W IV solution.

    _____ Vital signs must be taken every hour while a blood product is infusing.

    _____ Stay with the patient during the first 15 minutes of the infusion.

    _____ The infusion should run at 2 mL/min for the first 15 minutes.

    _____ Vital signs are taken every 30 minutes if they are stable after the first 15 minutes.

    _____ Two nurses must verify the donor number, patient ID number, patient name, and ABO and Rh type on the blood bag, on the patient's blood armband, and on the slip accompanying the unit.

7. What is the average infusion time for a unit of packed red cells?
   a. 30 minutes
   b. 1 hour
   c. 2 hours
   d. 4 hours

8. Each patient must be carefully monitored for a transfusion reaction. Signs and symptoms of such a reaction include which of the following? Select all that apply.

   _____ Chills

   _____ Fever

   _____ Stomach ache

   _____ Back pain

   _____ Cramps in the legs

   _____ Itching

   _____ Shortness of breath

   _____ Cough

9. What must be done immediately if a patient exhibits signs or symptoms of a transfusion reaction?

10. Most transfusion reactions occur during _____ of the infusion.

Care of the Surgical Patient: Pre- and Intraoperative Care

/♌ **Reading Assignment:** Care of the Surgical Patient (Chapter 37)

Patients: Piya Jordan, Medical-Surgical Floor, Room 403
Clarence Hughes, Medical-Surgical Floor, Room 404

Objectives:

1. Identify preoperative procedures necessary for the patient scheduled for surgery.
2. List measures to be carried out for the patient to be readied for surgery.
3. Discuss care in the postanesthesia care unit (PACU).
4. Identify necessary elements of the PACU report to the floor.

Exercise 1

 CD-ROM Activity—Preoperative Care

 30 minutes

- Sign in to work at Pacific View Regional Hospital on the Medical-Surgical Floor for Period of Care 1. (*Note:* If you are already in the virtual hospital from a previous exercise, click on **Leave the Floor** and then **Restart the Program** to get to the sign-in window.)
- From the Patient List, select Piya Jordan (Room 403).
- Click on **Get Report** and read the report.
- Click on **Go to Nurses' Station**.
- Click on **Chart** and then on **403**.
- Click on the **Surgical Reports** tab. Scroll to the Preoperative Patient Instruction Sheet.

1. What instructions regarding hygiene were given to Piya Jordan in preparation for her surgery?

2. What were the instructions regarding eating or drinking?

3. According to the surgical admission sheet, Piya Jordan was scheduled for a

_____.

Read in your medical-surgical textbook about colectomy.

4. What does a colectomy involve? Why is it being done in Piya Jordan's case? (*Hint:* Review the **History and Physical**.)

5. Which of the following risk factors for surgical complications apply to Piya Jordan? Select all that apply.

_____ Obesity

_____ Age

_____ Blood disorder

_____ Heart disease

_____ Respiratory disease

_____ Immune disorder

_____ Drug abuse

_____ Chronic pain

→ • Return to the **Surgical Reports** section of the chart. Scroll to the Surgery Procedures and Treatments form.

6. The preoperative sedation Piya Jordan received was _____.

Read in your pharmacology book or your nursing drug handbook about this medication.

7. Below, provide the requested information about the preoperative medication you provided in question 6.

Medication Order	Action	Onset and Duration

8. Before administering preoperative medications, what must be checked or done?

9. When the nurse was teaching Piya Jordan about the use of the incentive spirometer preoperatively, she should have told her to do what?
   a. Inhale through her nose.
   b. Complete five full breaths for each session.
   c. Inhale completely and hold for at least 3 seconds.
   d. Exhale completely and hold for at least 10 seconds.

10. From the following list, identify the tubes and devices that Piya Jordan was told will be in place postoperatively. Select all that apply.

   _____ Abdominal binder

   _____ IV

   _____ NG tube

   _____ Foley catheter

   _____ Sequential compression devices (SCDs)

   _____ Abduction wedge

   _____ Patient analgesia controller

   _____ J-P suction device with drain

   _____ Traction apparatus

Exercise 2

Writing Activity—Intraoperative and Postanesthesia Care

15 minutes

1. Piya Jordan received _____ anesthesia.

2. The roles of the scrub nurse and the circulating nurse vary. Below, identify which functions each nurse would perform.

Functions   **Nurse**

_____   Sets up the instruments   a. Circulating nurse

_____   Carries out the "time out" surgical site   b. Scrub nurse
        identification
                                                   c. Circulating nurse and scrub nurse
_____   Gowns and gloves the surgeon

_____   Points out breaks in sterile technique

_____   Counts sponges and instruments

_____   Hands instruments to the operating team

_____   Obtains needed fluids and medications

_____   Takes charge of tissue specimens

_____   Positions lights and stools

_____   Assists with gowning and gloving

_____   Checks function of each piece of equipment

_____   Verifies that the electric cautery is properly
        grounded

_____   Positions patient on the table and pads
        potential pressure areas

_____   Communicates with those outside the OR

3. The _____ monitors the patient's vital signs during the operation.

4. When surgery is over, the patient is moved to the postanesthesia care unit (PACU) and

   is positioned to _____ and

   _____.

5. In the PACU, the vital signs are measured and documented _____ until

   _____.

6. The Aldrete scoring system is often used to determine when the patient is ready for transfer back to the nursing unit. Below and on the next page, select each of the areas that is scored with this system. Select all that apply.

   _____   Time in PACU

   _____   Respiration

_____ Consciousness

_____ Gag reflex

_____ Skin color

_____ Circulation

_____ Activity

_____ Speech

7. Two important functions of the PACU nurse are to keep the patient _____

and to reassure the patient that _____.

8. Because Piya Jordan has preexisting atrial fibrillation, the PACU nurse will monitor her closely. What assessments should the nurse perform related to this problem? (*Hint:* Use critical thinking for this question.)

Exercise 3

CD-ROM Activity—Another Surgery

30 minutes

- Sign in to work at Pacific View Regional Hospital on the Medical-Surgical Floor for Period of Care 1. (*Note:* If you are already in the virtual hospital from a previous exercise, click on **Leave the Floor** and then **Restart the Program** to get to the sign-in window.)
- From the Patient List, select Clarence Hughes (Room 404).
- Click on **Get Report** and read the report.
- Click on **Go to Nurses' Station** and then on **404** to visit Clarence Hughes.
- Click on **Chart** and then on the chart for **404**. Click on the tab for **Surgical Reports**.

1. The surgical procedure that Clarence Hughes underwent was a _____

_____.

2. Preoperatively, the nurse verifies the disposition of Clarence Hughes' valuables. What does the preoperative form indicate as to the disposition of his valuables?

3. Because of the type of surgery Clarence Hughes had, he will not be able to exercise his foot and leg to the same extent that Piya Jordan is encouraged to do postoperatively. Thus he is at high risk for deep vein thrombosis. What would you encourage him to do with his lower left extremity?

4. What scheduled medications did the surgeon OK for Clarence Hughes to have in the immediate preoperative period?

5. Below, note the preoperative medication that Clarence Hughes received, along with the action, onset, and duration of each. (*Hint:* See the Drug Guide or check your pharmacology or nursing drug handbook.)

Preoperative Medication	Action	Onset and Duration

6. What procedures were performed on Clarence Hughes before his surgery was begun?

7. Clarence Hughes' surgery lasted _____.

8. What was tobramycin used for during this surgery?

9. What is in Clarence Hughes' history that makes it especially important for him to be diligent in using his incentive spirometer after surgery?

LESSON **21** ————————————————————

Care of the Surgical Patient: Postoperative Care

————————————————————————————————

Reading Assignment: Diet Therapy and Assisted Feeding (Chapter 27)
Care of the Surgical Patient (Chapter 37)
Providing Wound Care and Treating Pressure Ulcers
   (Chapter 38)
Promoting Musculoskeletal Function (Chapter 39)

Patients: Piya Jordan, Medical-Surgical Floor, Room 403
Clarence Hughes, Medical-Surgical Floor, Room 404
Kathryn Doyle, Skilled Nursing Floor, Room 503

Objectives:

1. Discuss necessary elements of the PACU report to the floor.
2. Identify assessments necessary for a patient returning to the nursing unit from surgery.
3. Prioritize care for the fresh postoperative patient.
4. Assist with convalescence and recovery after surgery.

Exercise 1

 CD-ROM Activity—Postoperative Care After Knee Replacement

 30 minutes

- Sign in to work at Pacific View Regional Hospital on the Medical-Surgical Floor for Period of Care 1. (*Note:* If you are already in the virtual hospital from a previous exercise, click on **Leave the Floor** and then **Restart the Program** to get to the sign-in window.)
- From the Patient List, select Clarence Hughes (Room 404).
- Click on **Go to Nurses' Station** and then on **Chart**.
- Select the chart for **404** and click on **Physician's Orders**. Review the postoperative orders for Clarence Hughes.

1. What is the purpose of continuous passive motion by machine after joint replacement surgery?

2. What would you do before placing Clarence Hughes' knee in the CPM machine?

3. What is the goal for angle of flexion for Clarence Hughes today, the second postoperative day? Would you set the machine for this goal degree when beginning the procedure for the day?

4. How would you determine how well Clarence Hughes is tolerating the CPM machine?

5. Clarence Hughes is to ambulate twice a day. He will initially use a walker to do this. You

   know that the walker height is appropriate for him if his elbows are bent _____ degrees when his hands are on the handgrips and he is standing upright.

6. When checking the walker for safety, you would check to see that the

   _____ on the legs are intact.

→ • Click on **Return to Nurses' Station** and then on **404**.
   • Inside the patient's room, click on **Patient Care** and then on **Chest**. From the list of assessment subcategories (the green boxes), choose **Respiratory** and perform a respiratory assessment.

7. Clarence Hughes is at high risk of respiratory complications because he is a smoker. Record your findings from his respiratory assessment below.

➤ • Now click on **EPR** and **Login**. Choose **404** as the Patient and **Respiratory** as the Category. Document your assessment findings from above.
   • Scroll back and review the previous respiratory findings review.

8. Has Clarence Hughes been using his incentive spirometer regularly?

9. Clarence Hughes is to use his incentive spirometer regularly. Check his orders and then decide which of the following teaching points you should go over with him. Select all that apply.

_____ Exhale through the nose.

_____ Inhale slowly and deeply.

_____ Hold the inhalation for 3 seconds.

_____ Use the spirometer for 20 breaths with each use.

_____ Make the ball rise to the marker with each inhalation.

_____ Breathe normally between each breath on the spirometer.

_____ Exhale into the spirometer forcefully.

_____ Use the spirometer ten times each hour while awake.

_____ Pucker lips when exhaling.

Exercise 2

 CD-ROM Activity—Care of the Postoperative Patient

 30 minutes

- Sign in to work at Pacific View Regional Hospital on the Medical-Surgical Floor for Period of Care 1. (*Note:* If you are already in the virtual hospital from a previous exercise, click on **Leave the Floor** and then **Restart the Program** to get to the sign-in window.)
- From the Patient List, select Piya Jordan (Room 403).
- Click on **Go to Nurses' Station**.
- Click on **Chart** and then on **403**. Select **Physician's Orders** and review the postoperative orders.

    1. After you receive a newly arrived postoperative patient and get report from the PACU nurse, what initial assessments would you make once the patient is settled in the unit?

    2. What is the schedule for frequent vital sign measurements for a patient who has just returned from the operating room?

    3. Piya Jordan needs to be repositioned every 2 hours. How can she be positioned after this surgery?

 - Click on **Return to Nurses' Station** and then on **403**.
- Click on **Patient Care** and then on **Abdomen**.

4. Piya Jordan had an exploratory laparotomy and right hemicolectomy. For this reason, an abdominal assessment is of high priority. Assess each aspect of the abdominal area and record the findings below. (*Hint:* To perform this assessment, click on each of the subcategories in the green boxes, as well as on the **Equipment** button to the right of the green boxes.)

Integumentary

Musculoskeletal

Gastrointestinal

Equipment

➡ • Now click on **EPR** and on **Login**. Select **403** in the Patient box and document your findings from Piya Jordan's abdominal assessment. To do so, you will need to access the **Gastrointestinal** and the **Wounds and Drains** flow charts, using the Category drop-down menu.

5. What effect may Piya Jordan's age have on her wound healing?

6. Piya Jordan is presently in the _____ stage of wound healing, which lasts

about _____ days.

7. Piya Jordan has a _____ wound drainage device.

8. What must be done after emptying the suction system in order to reactivate it?

9. Because Piya Jordan has had abdominal surgery, getting her to cough adequately will be difficult. Explain how you would prepare and assist her with coughing.

10. The physician has ordered sequential compression devices for Piya Jordan. What is the purpose of these devices?

11. Piya Jordan's physician has ordered KCl be added to her IV fluids during the postoperative period. What assessment parameter must be considered when administering KCl to the patient?
    a. Respiratory rate
    b. Blood pressure
    c. Heart rate
    d. Temperature
    e. Intake
    f. Output

Exercise 3

  CD-ROM Activity—Surgical Recovery and Medication Administration

30 minutes

Kathryn Doyle is in the Skilled Nursing Unit recovering from hip surgery.

- Sign in to work at Pacific View Regional Hospital on the Skilled Nursing Floor for Period of Care 1. (*Note:* If you are already in the virtual hospital from a previous exercise, click on **Leave the Floor** and then **Restart the Program** to get to the sign-in window.)
- From the Patient List, select Kathryn Doyle (Room 503).
- Click on **Get Report** and read the report.
- Click on **Go to Nurses' Station** and then on **503**. Read the **Initial Observations**.

  1. Kathryn Doyle has dry mucous membranes, which could indicate _____.

- Click on **Take Vital Signs**.

  2. Record Kathryn Doyle's current vital signs below.

     BP _____ SpO$_2$ _____ T _____ HR _____ RR _____ Pain _____

- Click on **Patient Care** and perform a focused assessment on Kathryn Doyle, particularly looking for potential surgical complications.

  3. What abnormalities did you find during the respiratory assessment for Kathryn Doyle?

  4. What interventions can be implemented for Kathryn Doyle to improve her respiratory function?

  5. Kathryn Doyle's Homans' sign was _____, and there is no evidence of

     the vascular complication of _____.

- Click on **MAR** and see what medications are scheduled for Kathryn Doyle at 0800.

6. Below, list the medications you are to administer to Kathryn Doyle. For each, provide the classification and its action or the reason for giving it.

Medication Order	Classification	Action/Reason for Administration

- Click on **Medication Room** on the bottom of your screen and begin to prepare Kathryn Doyle's 0800 medications.
- Click on **Unit Dosage** or on the unit dosage cart. Select drawer **503**.
- Using the Five Rights and the Five Responsibilities, follow the onscreen steps to select the 0800 medications for Kathryn Doyle. For each selection, click on **Put Medication on Tray**.

7. In comparison with the orders, were there any problems with the medications that were in the drawer?

8. What should you do?

• When all of the 0800 medications are on the tray, click on **Close Drawer**. Next, click **Review Medications**, performing the second check for each dose ordered for 0800.

- Click **Return to Medication Room** and then on **View Medication Room**.

- Click on **Preparation** or on the tray on the left side of your screen.

- For each medication, click on **Prepare** and provide the information requested by the Preparation Wizard.

- When all medications have been prepared, click on **Finish** and then on **Return to Medication Room**.

- Click on **503** to return to the patient's room. Click on **Patient Care** and then on **Medication Administration**.

- Administer each medication by clicking the down arrow next to **Select**, choosing **Administer** and following the prompts.

- When you have finished the 0800 medication administration, click on **Leave the Floor** and then on **Look at Your Preceptor's Evaluation**. Click on **Medication Scorecard** to see how you did.

9. What three things should you have done before you rechecked and opened the medication unit dose packages?